Building

Left-Brain
Power

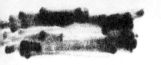

ALSO BY THE AUTHORS:

Brain-Building Games
Building Mental Muscle
Exercises for the Whole Brain
How Sharp Is Your Pencil?
Right-Brain Teasers
Use It or Lose It!

Building
Left-Brain
Power

Allen D. Bragdon

and

David Gamon, Ph.D.

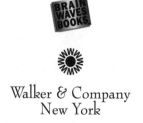

Walker & Company
New York

First published in the United States of America by Allen D. Bragdon Publishers, Inc.
BRAINWAVES® is a registered trademark of Allen D. Bragdon Publishers Inc.
This edition published by Walker Publishing Company, Inc.

Published simultaneously in Canada by Fitzhenry and Whiteside,
Markham, Ontario L3R 4T8

For information about permission to reproduce selections from this book,
write to Permissions, Walker & Company, 104 Fifth Avenue,
New York, New York 10011

Library of Congress Cataloging-in-Publication Data available upon request

ISBN 0-8027-7683-3

Visit Walker & Company's Web site at www.walkerbooks.com

Printed in the United States of America

2   4   6   8   10   9   7   5   3

*The brain has muscles for thinking
as the legs have muscles for walking.*
— J. O. De La Mettrie: *L'Homme machine*, 1748

Use it or lose it.
— Tallulah Bankhead, Actress, circa. 1950
(Attributed: with reference, perhaps, to the functions of
different but equally delightful systems)

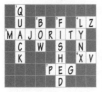
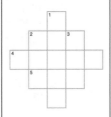

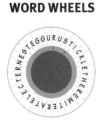

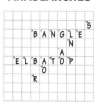
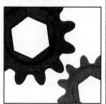

HOW THE LEFT SIDE OF YOUR BRAIN WORKS FOR YOU

T his book is the second in the new Brainwaves® series. Like the first, *Building Mental Muscle,* this book offers synopses of current brain research that can be practically applied to real-word situations. The interactive exercises provide opportunities to apply the research findings and, simultaneously, to stimulate and strengthen targeted skills controlled by the left hemisphere of the brain. Recent invention of technologies to measure how the brain works have released a torrent of research on how learning takes place. This is proving that the "Use It or Lose It" principle applies to our brains as well as our biceps, and that idle brain cells can be re-activated by enticing them to go back to work.

The left hemisphere evolved to draw comparisons between new incoming data and old data already known

Moreover it arranges abstract symbols into patterns that represent reality. This equips the brain to plan ahead by visualizing the future. ("Six coins this size and five that size would buy a nanny goat whose milk will make enough cheese to buy another nanny goat three moons from now.") It allows people to agree that certain sounds and marks can be strung together to describe what happened somewhere else at some other time. ("Language saves time. Now I can walk over the mountain and tell the other tribe: 'Big flood yesterday. Many fish.' Otherwise, I'd have to to drag all of them over to my side of the mountain and point to the mess.")

And, best of all, *your left brain LOVES its job!*

Back in the early 1960's a research team at the University of California, Berkeley led by Mark Rosenzweig and Marion Diamond took a few of their genetically identical, very young, lab mice out of their comfortable cages and put them into much larger comfortable cages. They left other mice of the same age alone in their smaller cages. Every few days they put another new piece of tiny mouse-gym equipment into the larger cages — running wheels, tunnels, climbing platforms and such. Both groups of mice had a great life with plenty of food and water and clean cages. But the "enriched environment" group that got lots of new stuff to figure out and play with every day were constantly experimenting and always actively engaged.

After several weeks, well through adolescence in mouse-time, the brains of all the mice in the old and new test cages were measured, weighed and compared. As predicted, Rosenzweig and Diamond found that the brains of the mice with the frequent new challenges to meet had grown heavier and had more connections, with higher levels of neurotransmitters to stimulate or inhibit mental activity. The researchers couldn't tell which group was *happier,* but the challenged group certainly didn't lie around looking bored. They were all over their toys all the time inventing ways to use them. That mental activity constantly stimulated the development of new cells in their young brains and provided increased physical exercise, which also stimulates brain growth.

What's more, the research group at U.C. Berkeley and later a research team at the University of Illinois, confirmed that mentally active mice not only grew brains more densely packed with neurons but also took less time to solve problems such as learning how to find their way through a maze. Of course, they were only mice but it is amazing how little human DNA differs from a mouse's. And, *vive la différence!* Most of the difference between the human brain and the brains of other animals which have evolved along different lines — those uniquely human skills that include language, math, conscious recall of past data to plan future goals — are processed in the *left* hemisphere and pre-frontal areas.

Popular myths about brains are contradicted by research

Until very recently, the accepted dogma in the brain sciences has been that, once you're born, all your brain has to look forward to is a long and steady loss of brain cells (also known as *neurons*). Many of life's little events, routine and otherwise — mini-strokes, drinking a glass of wine, holding your breath, the very fact of living — would pick off the neurons in your cerebral cortex like ducks in a shooting gallery. And, it was also once thought, no new brain cells would grow to take the place of the extinguished ones, since nerve cells in your brain and spinal cord could not regenerate. But current research is showing clear evidence that "stem" cells in the human brain *can* create new neurons and that relatively idle neurons will begin to extend their branches to carry signals to and from other neurons.

Even the widespread belief that we use only a tiny fraction of our brains has never been supported by facts. It's a bit of a mystery how the idea took hold in popular culture in the first place. As neurologist Oliver Sacks points out, the brain is an organ that uses a lot of energy and a lot of blood. Our bodies simply can't afford the luxury of allowing large unused portions of any organ to continue to draw off energy from the body's limited supply of nutrients in the blood. If neurons dedicated to perform a given skill are not being used they will either atrophy or be co-opted to some other function.

Through all the debates about the respective roles of nature and nurture in shaping human behavior, the notion has persisted that intelligence is fixed from birth. If we really believe this, it might not matter what we do with the brain we're born with, since (according to folk wisdom) nothing can change the inherent abilities and limitations with which our genes endow us. But it *does* matter. Everyone knows the brain can acquire facts. The good news is that we can sharpen our ability to sort them, interpret them and use these facts. In other words...

Uncultivated mental skills can be regained with use

Outdated beliefs have helped make us complacent about our brains. We spend huge amounts of money and time keeping our bodies in shape at health clubs, but how much time is spent on mental fitness? When we retire, we imagine that it's our just reward to rid our lives of all mental challenge. And yet, anybody who's had a friend or family member succumb to Alzheimer's knows that an active brain contributes to the quality of life.

When the infant laboratory animals described above were exposed to an enriched environment of lots of playmates and toys, the extra stimulation literally made their brains larger and their neurons send out more and longer branches, called *axons* and *dendrites*. In fact, mice in the enriched environment showed an increase of 4000 new neurons in the hippocampus compared to 2400 in the control group without toys and playmates. This fit well with existing research showing that young brains can call on a large bank of neurons to start filling the need to develop new skills. What surprised the researchers was that the same results occurred when *old* mice (three years is old for mice) were transferred from a life-long impoverished environment to an enriched one. Their brains got bigger and better, too, and quite quickly in fact, just as elderly people who begin to exercise can rebuild muscle mass surprisingly quickly.

These findings have been known in the research community for many years, and yet very few laypeople are familiar with them. They point to a very important conclusion. We may have been misguided all along in our preoccupation with the *number* of neurons in our brains. More important than number may be the *quality* of our brain cells. Simply put, a higher-quality brain cell is one that has a rich system of dendrites reaching out to make contact with other brain cells. Diamond and Rosenzweig's work showed that challenging mental exercise and social contact can

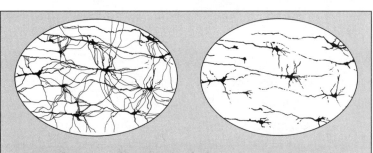

Active brain cells, above left, create richer networks of interconnecting dendrites and axons than do cells allowed to remain idle, shown right. When stimulated, idle cells create branches to process complex mental tasks efficiently.

give even older mice bigger, better brains by improving brain cell quality even if not quantity.

More recent work has shown that improved neuron quality may not be the only reason brains can get bigger and better late in life. Two bodies of independent research reported in March 1999, out of the Salk Institute in San Diego and Princeton University, add to other new evidence that adult animals do indeed grow new brain cells. (A Purdue researcher, Joseph Altman, actually offered evidence for this 30 years ago, but most scientists simply dismissed his findings.) Even more exciting are the factors that the studies show for promoting such growth. In the Salk study, mice that exercised regularly on a running wheel grew twice as many new brain cells as other mice. The new cells appeared in the hippocampus, a part of the brain crucial for memory and learning. In the Princeton study, led by psychologist Elizabeth Gould, the apparent cause of the mice's doubled brain-cell growth was *mental* exercise. Her research proved that challenging mental tasks not only spurred the production of new hippocampal brain cells, but helped maintain existing ones. As Gould herself put it, "It's a classic case of 'use it or lose it.'"

Since you're not a laboratory mouse do these findings apply to you?

A Swedish-American team led by the Salk Institute's Fred Gage recently found that adult human brains can and do grow new neurons throughout life. This fits well with another recent study of U.C. Berkeley professors which showed that cognitive abilities that usually decline with age — planning, organizing, and manipulating new information in terms of prior knowledge — are preserved in older professors who continue to challenge themselves with demanding intellectual activity.

So it's time we accepted the fact that one of the most fundamental claims of 20th-century brain science — that adult brains can't grow new neurons — is false. Adult brains *do* grow more new brain cells and connections between existing cells in several ways. One is physical exercise. Another is good diet. Another is to enrich your environment with social contact and mental activities that are both fun and challenging.

Common misunderstandings about the "good" right hemisphere and the "bad" left hemisphere

In the late 1970's, art teacher Betty Edwards wrote a very popular book called *Drawing on the Right Side of the Brain* that was based on her experiences with young art students. Her "right-brain" approach to teaching how to draw an accurate likeness emphasized learning to see the whole form rather than focusing on component parts, and on learning to render *literally* what you see by ignoring the left-brain's tendency to view a subject in terms of what it has seen before. One of Ms. Edwards' tricks to help students do this was to turn a photo upside-down before drawing it. This trick encouraged the untrained artist to allow the "literal" right brain to view, say, eye glasses seen from the side, as oval shapes and prevented the left hemisphere from "seeing" them as idealized eye glasses with round lenses. Many people who were influenced by such art instruction techniques came to think of artistic, holistic, or spiritual people as "right-brained," or as "left-brained" if they were practical, logical or unimaginative.

But, brain researchers began to point out that the human brain cannot be divided up neatly, or even roughly, along those lines. In fact, some stereotypically male skills, such as the spatial visualization involved in, say, map-reading or construction, are more right- than left-brain, while some "female" ones such as verbal skill are predominantly left-brain. Musical skills are distributed across both hemispheres, with more left-brain involvement as the skill level rises. Current brain research clearly shows how interconnected our internal neuronal ecosystem is and how wrong it is to claim that a single label such as "female" or even "music" matches up with a single part of the brain.

The "happier" hemisphere. Recent research reveals how left vs. right hemisphere dominance affects mood

For a long time, neurologists and other medical practitioners have noted that people who have suffered damage only to the right side of their brains — whether caused by stroke, tumor, or injury — tend to suffer from depression. Something in their left hemisphere, then, must help to maintain a happy, motivated outlook on life. As far back as 1982 Harold Sackheim's research, based on observations of patients with emotional disorders arising from brain injury or disease, posited a right-hemisphere specialization for crying, and a left-hemisphere specialization for laughing.

More recent studies using brain imaging technology have confirmed the left brain's role in positive emotions, and the right's involvement in negative emotions. PET scans show that the front part of the right hemisphere is activated when a person feels negative emotions, such as depression, fear, disgust, or anger, and many depressed patients have overactive regions in the right front part of their brain. Breakthrough research by leading neuroscientists including Drevets and Damasio, clearly reveals that a depressed mood is associated with *under*activity in prefrontal regions of the left hemisphere. If the same area is *over*active, the result may be extreme happiness, even mania. Most people feel a sense of positive satisfaction when their left brain is busy.

More recent studies by Australian researcher Jack Pettigrew at the University of Brisbane, propose a "sticky switch" explanation for bipolar disorder, also known as manic depression. Normally, humans process positive emotions in the left hemisphere, and negative ones in the right. Normally, too, the two hemispheres constantly exchange impulses at a high rate of speed. Thus, we can feel a mix of emotions or have good or bad moods, as some mechanism in our brain switches activity from one hemisphere to the other. What makes bipolar patients different is that their switch is slow, and tends to get stuck in one setting or the other. When the switch is stuck in the left-hemisphere setting, the patients are manic; when it's stuck in the right-hemisphere setting, they're depressed.

The two domains are mutually reinforcing, with each hemisphere's specializations helping the other's to develop. As brain researcher Robert Ornstein has put it in a recent book, "The right-hemisphere specializations develop to their fullest when informed by a fully developed left side." Conversely, of course, you don't help a child to learn how to read by denying her the opportunity to express her creativity.

What happens if the right and left sides of the brain can no longer communicate to each other what they know?
Dramatic insights into differences between the left and right hemispheres have come from studies of people who've had the

neurons that connect the right and left sides, or hemispheres, of their brain severed. This operation splits the brain into two independent halves by cutting through the *corpus callosum,* the main bundle of nerves binding the brain's left and right hemispheres together. Doctors started performing these split-brain operations in the 1940s to reduce the severity of epileptic seizures by preventing a seizure that starts on one side from spreading to the other side of the brain. Oddly, such split-brain patients appear to function like everybody else, moving normally through everyday lives — until their behavior is examined closely and tested professionally. For example: medical literature tells of a split-brain patient whose two hands (each of which is controlled by a different hemisphere) fought with each other while he was getting dressed in the morning. One hand would try to pull on the pants while the other struggled to pull them off. Another patient was awakened by a hand — her own — slapping her across the face. The half of her brain controlling that hand had woken up, realized the other half of the brain was oversleeping, and decided to remedy the situation.

Since each half of the brain controls the opposite side of the body's movements and sensations, a split-brain patient who is holding a pencil out of his own sight in his *left* hand receives that information with his *right* brain. Because his corpus callosum is severed, the right side of his brain can't communicate with the left. Since the left brain commonly controls speech, he simply can't tell you the fact that he has a pencil in his left hand.

The right side of his brain knows the pencil is in his left hand, even if the left does not. If you then show him a selection of pictures, and ask him to point out the object he'd been holding in his hand, his *left* hand will point to a picture of a pencil. This tips off the left brain *visually* where the pencil is, so it can now tell you in words what the right brain knew but couldn't say.

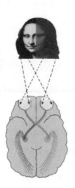

Your eyes, unlike your hands and feet, are not linked simply to the opposite brain hemisphere. Each eye sends information to both hemispheres: for each eye, things you see in the left of your visual field (to the left of your nose if you're looking straight ahead) are conveyed to your right brain, while your right visual field connects to your left brain. Normally, both brain hemispheres get information from the whole field since they're in constant communication with each other.

Focus your eyes on the nose of the split-face chimera to the right. Quick, which impression is stronger? The woman or the man? If the woman, your right hemisphere is dominating; if the man, your left hemisphere has taken over. (Under laboratory conditions researchers ask the subject to focus on a dot in the center of a screen onto which they quickly flash the split-face picture.)

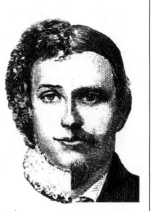

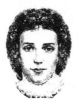

If the two sides of your brain couldn't talk to each other across your corpus callosum, your right brain would have seen only the woman, the left brain would only have seen the man. If you were then shown these full-face pictures and asked which picture you'd just seen, you'd answer, "The man." But if asked to point out with your left hand what you'd just seen, you'd point to the woman. And if then asked why you were pointing to the woman, your left brain would fabricate an excuse such as, "I really meant to point to the man, my hand slipped."

Even though communication from one side of your brain to the other across your corpus callosum is virtually instantaneous, it isn't perfect. The brain hemisphere that gets information directly from your senses has an advantage over the one that gets it indirectly across the corpus callosum. In carefully designed experiments, it's easier to read written words flashed to the right visual field, connecting directly to the left hemisphere. On the other hand, faces are easier to recognize when flashed to the left visual field. Also, each one of your ears sends information to both brain hemispheres, but cross-connections from left ear to right brain, or right ear to left brain are stronger than same-side connections. The difference is unimportant except when there's competition for access to your left-hemisphere language centers. For example, when you're trying to listen to a single voice in a noisy bar you might unconsciously tilt your head so that you listen with your right ear. You can try a simple experiment right now to test the hypothesis that you'll favor your right ear for sounds that are hard to hear. Pretend that you want to eavesdrop on a conversation on the other side of a wall. When you approach the wall, which ear do you press against it?

You may not be able to feel it happening, but while you are engaging in the following tasks, activity will be increasing in either your left or your right hemisphere

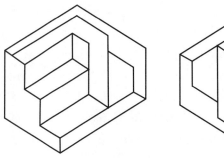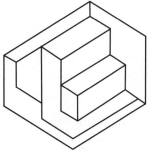

What is odd about the shapes shown on the preceding page? The kind of task, that requires you to rotate or manipulate visual figures in your mind's eye is typical of the sort of test designed to gauge your visual or spatial intelligence. One reason puzzles like these serve well to isolate right-brain visual skills is that it's virtually impossible to translate them into a verbal mode. The demands placed on your brain are about as purely visual as you can get, unlike, say, the demands made by a spatial task requiring metric distance judgments, and you can therefore be sure that people who are good at tasks like these aren't falling back on their language skills to get themselves to the right answer.

Next, take a look at the pairs of words below, another game similar to what you'll find on some standard intelligence-test batteries. Here, the trick is to figure out what features the paired words have in common.

Tree - Fly
Orange - Banana
Happiness - Anger
Praise - Punishment
Hammer - Screwdriver
Promise - Disappointment

It makes sense that the sort of reasoning involved here would be left-brain because it is language-based. The parallel concepts are not visual; the similarities have little to do with what the meaning of the word *looks* like. They are related to function or are abstractly symbolic, so it would be very difficult to express what the similarities are in anything other than words. Studies of split-brain patients and of stroke patients, as well as PET scan studies of "normal" brains, back up the hypothesis that tasks like these typically involve the left hemisphere far more than the right.

The right and left hemispheres offer different strategies for solving problems, and cooperate in that endeavor, though one side may be more specialized in a given skill

To get an idea how different strategies can be applied to yield possibly different results, examine the photo below. It is a painting by the 16th-century Milanese artist Giuseppe Arcimboldo. What do you see? A face? Lots of fish? Of course, you can see either, and you can switch rapidly back and forth between the two. Like "the

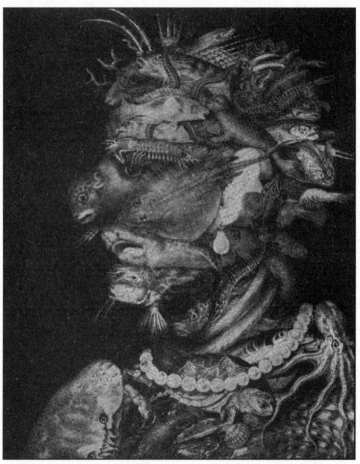

Split-brain patients presented with this picture in their left visual field (connecting to the right hemisphere) see only the face; in their right visual field (left hemisphere), they see only fish.

forest or the trees" the difference corresponds to a left-brain vs. right-brain approach.

It's not so much that a well-developed left hemisphere interferes with the full development of the right brain, or that the left and right hemispheres are antagonists in a competition for finite resources or energy allocations. All our brain's skills are valuable and mutually supporting. To the extent that they can be viewed separately, the two hemispheres give us different perspectives to problems and offer complementary approaches to solve them. Sometimes, a sequential, verbal, linear approach works best; other times, a configurational or visually-based strategy might point to the best results.

Why are the uniquely human skills monitored by the left-hemisphere worth building up?

In brief, there are three reasons: those skills improve career opportunity, emotional outlook and quality of life in later years. Noted neuroscientist Michael Gazzaniga goes so far as to assert that "years of split-brain research informs us that the left hemisphere has many more mental capacities than the right. The right hemisphere's level of awareness is limited; it knows precious little about a lot of things." Most researchers would concede that the sorts of abilities housed in the left brain — analytical problem-solving, language, computational skills, logic — are ones that most people think of as demonstrations of intelligence. In fact, they largely define what it means to be human.

Left-brain injuries tend to destroy speech, a skill loss that can be easily and dramatically observed. Curiously, injuries to the right hemisphere tend to be ignored or belittled by those who suffer them even though they produce irrational, anti-social behavior bordering on monomania. President Woodrow Wilson continued several years in office after a right-brain stroke. The highly-respected Justice William O. Douglas also suffered serious stroke-damage to his right hemisphere, but continued to participate in the deliberations of the Supreme Court for months, unaware of his cognitive limitations and dismissing the paralysis of the left side of his body. In both cases the right-hemisphere damage had spared their speech but no longer enabled them to update their self-awareness. And here's bad news for men: they suffer more left-hemisphere strokes than women do, in general, and take longer to recover speech afterward. One reason for their slower recovery is that men tend to be more right-hemisphere specialized and the corpus collusum fibers connecting their two hemispheres are not as dense as women's are. Hence, women can more easily transfer language functions from damaged areas in the left side to their undamaged right side. However, differences in hemisphere dominance are generally more pronounced between left-handed people and right-handed people than they are between the sexes.

Left-brain skills tend to be identified with competence in professional and academic pursuits
Carl Sagan identified human, right-brain abilities as those we share with other animals, and left brain skills as those that tend to be more specific to our species. That is one reason why it may be that left-brain subjects are stressed in our educational system. Left-brain skills are also less "intuitive" than the crisis-management reaction to new data that the right hemisphere is set up to trigger. But your left side is fiercely determined to seek out how newly-introduced data may share *something* in common with other discreet data it has already composed into meaningful arrays. It is a great tool for spotting trends, solving algebra problems and composing clear, step-by-step instructions for assembling a barbecue grill — the skills that must be learned and practiced in order to succeed.

Demands placed on you may shift with time or circumstance, so it's good to have many strategies at your disposal to deal with new challenges that may arise. Whether you do or don't criticize teenagers for larding their speech with such imprecise colloquialisms as "you know" and "I'm, like, I dunno!", the inescapable fact is that most people need logical thinking and the ability to express themselves precisely to get and hold a job and maintain their professional edge. The fact that people do have an understanding, in a face-to-face interaction at least, of what a teenager means when she says, And "I was all, like, [facial expression]", doesn't mean that she can get away with that kind of language when she's delivering a report at a staff meeting or writing one up afterward.

The happy jolt-of-recognition that comes from suddenly realizing just how This-is-like-That! ranks high among the joys given to humankind

Those who protest that they're just not good at math or writing are suffering not so much from innate disability as from negative attitude and habit. The Germans have the word *Funktionslust* (pronounce it aloud for full impact) to refer to the kind of pleasure you get from doing something you're good at. For your pet cat, that pleasure may come from hunting voles on a warm summer night. For you, with your multitalented brain, with all your neural redundancies and your lack of hard-wired instinctual commitment to one specific task or one specific strategy, does pleasure come from otherwise complex hunting expeditions — hunting for an answer to a crossword puzzle clue, for example? To make the most of the mental capabilities you were born with you need to exercise them all. That is why this book presents such a wide variety of exercise formats targeted to specific mental skills.

Since either kind of hunt may require learned strategies

to get the prey, we've taken pains to try and clearly describe the techniques you may need to work out the exercises in this book. You may well find better ones. Our goal is to give you a taste of success. Most of us don't tackle new, potentially rewarding activities because there's nobody around to show us how easy it is to be good at them. If the only approach available is trial and error the left-brain skills you were born with are completely wasted. Everyone has heard of the notion that if a hundred monkeys poke randomly at the keys of a hundred typewriters, sooner or later one of those monkeys will come up with the complete works of William Shakespeare. Random trial and error can eventually lead to the right answer, but it's not very satisfying. Also it takes too long to come up with an answer to be competitive with problem-solving strategies your left hemisphere can cook up.

How this book is organized

You can dive into this book anywhere. You needn't read it from beginning to end. Everybody's mind works differently, but most people will find that the formats of the exercises in the chapters toward the beginning of the book are easier to solve than the ones near the end. Within each chapter the exercises progress from easier to harder, as shown by the thermometer-like difficulty scale at the top of each right-hand page.

A wide range of exercise formats maximize the excitement of acquiring new skills and honing old ones

Easier puzzles are at the beginning because we know how frustrating it can be to dive into a difficult puzzle in an unfamiliar format. Our goal is to get you started working in an unfamiliar skill area and allow your own sense of satisfaction take over as you begin to master it. The left brain excels not so much at sorting through completely new information, but at applying well-practiced, routinized codes and strategies in a quick and efficient way. But first, you have to learn the routine. (One major aspect of what's called "intelligence" reduces to nothing more than this kind of familiarity, developed through practice.) We've tried to set things up so this learning process will be maximally enjoyable and minimally frustrating.

Instructions on how to solve each of the 14 different exercise formats make new challenges manageable

At the beginning of each chapter, you'll find an explanation of how that specifically targeted mental exercise works and demonstrates strategies for solving them. In these chapter introductions, you'll also find interesting facts about the parts of your brain you'll be challenging when you work on the exercises.

Some exercise formats provide clues as crossword puzzles do. To help you get started if you're stuck, an optional "Starter" will help with strategies. For further help getting started (with an interlocking exercise especially), a small piece of the answer appears in a hint. We have made these hints particularly easy to ignore by printing them in small type, upside-down at the bottom of the page. The full solution to each exercise appears in the back of the book.

We have also included a test in some of the chapters. You can try them by yourself or with another person to take the measure of a skill related to the subject of the chapter. Some measure aptitudes and some temperament.

Information on how your brain solves problems and learns new techniques is written in non-technical language

The "Brain Bite" you'll find in almost every puzzle gives you a nugget of interesting information about the left hemisphere's skills and abilities, or about left-and-right-hemisphere differences. Often, this information is drawn from research reported in academic and scientific journals that we've listed in the reference section at the back of the book. That way, if you want to learn more, you can match the name of the researcher cited in the Brain Bite to an entry in the reference section, and look up the primary source.

Everybody's stupid at something. Try the exercises you think you will enjoy most, but sneak a look at the others
Everybody's brain is different, as are everybody's skills and abilities. The person who shies away from the word-skill exercises in the "Analock" chapter may have an easy time with "Codebreakers," while the relative difficulty may be reversed for someone else. We hope, though, that you will take advantage of this opportunity to sneak a look at the stuff you don't think you're good at. We all have a tendency to settle into fixed patterns of behavior, either out of laziness, fear of failure or habit. Problem-solving strategies can be learned and reinforced through practice. The broad array of exercises in this book lets you get started stimulating some of your precious, though temporarily idle neurons. The process is really quite a lot of fun, the hints and starters are there to give you a boost, and the solutions are in the back.

We hope your left hemisphere will thrive on the diverse engagements we have devised for it in the following pages. And, when you have worked out a solution to an exercise that looked daunting at first, we hope you will savor the private kind of joy that comes from applying your mental tools effectively to complete an unfamiliar task.

By ringing small changes on the words leg-of-mutton *and* turnip — *changes so gradual as to escape detection — I could "demonstrate" that a turnip was, is, and of right, ought to be a leg-of-mutton.*

Edgar Allan Poe, *Marginalia*, 1844-49

¹T	²H	³R	⁴O	⁵W
²H				E
³R				N
⁴O				D
⁵W	E	N	D	S

ANALOCKS

7 Anagramatic Manipulations
Self-Test: *Man or Woman?*

21

All about

ANALOCKS

Analock puzzles involve anagrams, which are letters that must be rearranged to form a real English word. (Sometimes you're given a regular word to start with, sometimes a nonsensical jumble.) What makes an Analock different from a typical anagram is that you write the answer both vertically and horizontally into a grid of letters intersecting with other answers. That gives you extra help solving each anagram, since the intersecting letters will fill in part of the solution to another anagram in the group. You're also given clues to the intended solution to each jumble.

Analocks are the first puzzle category in this book since from the solver's perspective they're one of the easiest. For a harder challenge, try your hand at *composing* an Analock. For example, try completing the one started on the facing page after you have solved some on the following pages. The intersecting format, which helps you deduce the solution to the puzzle, poses a challenge from the composer's point of view. Conversely, some of the most difficult puzzles to solve (the Codebreaker puzzles in the final chapter, for example) are the *easiest* to compose.

In a way, this somewhat paradoxical fact parallels some interesting facts about language itself. An infant confronting a jumble of arbitrary sounds is faced with the task of interpreting those sounds as discrete symbols, and then sorting those symbols into meaningful patterns of meaningful elements. The more built-in constraints that exist in the infant's brain about what might count as a "possible solution" to the puzzle of language acquisition, the easier the puzzle will presumably be for the infant to solve. But just think of the countless millennia of painstaking natural selection required to create those built-in constraints in the first place.

ANALOCK 1

1	2	3	4	5
2				
3				
4				
5				

Rearrange each group of capital letters to form a word (or a different word). Place the new word in the grid, starting in its numbered square, so that each word reads the same across or down. To make this exercise more difficult do not look at the "Starters" paragraph below. It contains clues to the correct words to make from all the anagrams. The upside-down "Hint" at the very bottom of this page gives the correct answer to one of the anagram words.

1. SVAEH   3. TAVER
2. NVAEH   4. SERVE
5. TERNE

Starters: These clues may help find the correct word hidden in each numbered anagram above: 1. Scrape 2. Safe place 3. Avoid 4. Poetry 5. Welcome sign

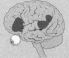

BRAIN BITES

Even though most right-handers (especially right-handed men) have their language centers in their left-brain, left-handedness isn't as good a predictor of right-brain language centers. Lorin Elias and M. P. Bryden found that *footedness* — which foot you use to kick or stomp — is a better predictor. So, by their studies, if you're left-footed, chances are good your language centers will be on the right side of your brain.

1	2	3	4	5
2				
3				
4				
5				

Rearrange each group of capital letters to form a word (or a different word). Place the new word in the grid, starting in its numbered square, so that each word reads the same across or down. To make this exercise more difficult do not look at the "Starters" paragraph below. It contains clues to the correct words to make from all the anagrams. The upside-down "Hint" at the very bottom of this page gives the correct answer to one of the anagram words.

1. STIVI   3. LYLIS
2. ISHIR   4. MISLA
5. METHY

Starters: These clues may help find the correct word hidden in each numbered anagram above: 1. Temporary stay 2. A Celtish nationality 3. Inane 4. Religious faith 5. Herb

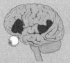

BRAIN BITES

C. Chiarello has found that the left hemisphere excels at rapid, automatic processing of printed words. The right hemisphere takes a less efficient, letter by letter approach, which may come in handy when the typeface or word shapes have unfamiliar forms.

1	2	3	4	5
2				
3				
4				
5				

Rearrange each group of capital letters to form a word (or a different word). Place the new word in the grid, starting in its numbered square, so that each word reads the same across or down. To make this exercise more difficult do not look at the "Starters" paragraph below. It contains clues to the correct words to make from all the anagrams. The upside-down "Hint" at the very bottom of this page gives the correct answer to one of the anagram words.

1. **RATTS**   3. **BODEA**

2. **OBART**   4. **INDOR**

5. **DRETN**

Starters: These clues may help find the correct word hidden in each numbered anagram above: 1. Initiate 2. Drum
3. Residence 4. Thinker maker 5. Tendency

BRAIN BITES

Why is language in the left hemisphere? The brain's right hemisphere is involved in early, less detailed stages of processing, which may also be those that emerge first in an infant's cognitive development. That may leave the left hemisphere available to specialize in more advanced operations on more detailed features, as in the kind of processing language skills involve.

1	2	3	4	5
2				
3				
4				
5				

Rearrange each group of capital letters to form a word (or a different word). Place the new word in the grid, starting in its numbered square, so that each word reads the same across or down. To make this exercise more difficult do not look at the "Starters" paragraph below. It contains clues to the correct words to make from all the anagrams. The upside-down "Hint" at the very bottom of this page gives the correct answer to one of the anagram words.

1. **PALAT**   3. **APAGE**

2. **GALLE**   4. **PRIAT**

5. **REALT**

Starters: These clues may help find the correct word hidden in each numbered anagram above: 1. Argentine silver, or river 2. Lawful 3. Open-mouthed 4. Pig-like mammal 5. Watchful

BRAIN BITES

Left-handers are quicker than right-handers at recovering their language abilities after a left-brain stroke — even those lefties who are left-hemisphere-dominant for language. That may mean that even left-handers with left-brain language centers are more likely to have passive right-brain language centers held in reserve, which may be activated should the need arise.

HINT: 1 = PLATA.

1	2	3	4	5
2				
3				
4				
5				

Rearrange each group of capital letters to form a word (or a different word). Place the new word in the grid, starting in its numbered square, so that each word reads the same across or down. To make this exercise more difficult do not look at the "Starters" paragraph below. It contains clues to the correct words to make from all the anagrams. The upside-down "Hint" at the very bottom of this page gives the correct answer to one of the anagram words.

1. **RESET**   3. **STERN**

2. **RESET**   4. **STERN**

5. **TRESS**

Starters: These clues may help find the correct word hidden in each numbered anagram above: 1. Chemical compound 2. Cubic meter 3. Sets of three 4. Max ___, painter 5. Musical signs

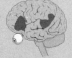

BRAIN BITES

Most left-handers still have language controlled at least partly by their left hemisphere. But left-handers with brain damage early in life are three times as likely to have right-brain language centers than other lefties. Paul Satz has proposed that impaired visuospatial abilities among left-handers with right-hemisphere speech may be due to their language centers displacing their right-brain spatial centers.

HINT: 2 = STERE.

	1	2	3	4	5
2					
3					
4					
5					

Rearrange each group of capital letters to form a word (or a different word). Place the new word in the grid, starting in its numbered square, so that each word reads the same across or down. To make this exercise more difficult do not look at the "Starters" paragraph below. It contains clues to the correct words to make from all the anagrams. The upside-down "Hint" at the very bottom of this page gives the correct answer to one of the anagram words.

1. CRUET   3. VAUUL
2. VIRRE   4. LESCL
5. ASEER

Starters: These clues may help find the correct word hidden in each numbered anagram above: 1. Armistice 2. Stream 3. Palate part 4. Electrolyte holders 5. Obliterate

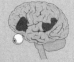

B R A I N B I T E S

On rare occasions, a brain tumor requires the removal of the dominant speech hemisphere (usually, the left). In young children, the remaining hemisphere can easily take over language abilities. Neuropsychologist Aaron Smith reports that even some adults make a reasonable recovery, although their sentences may remain relatively short and simple.

HINT: 3 = UVULA.

1	2	3	4	5
2				
3				
4				
5				

Rearrange each group of capital letters to form a word (or a different word). Place the new word in the grid, starting in its numbered square, so that each word reads the same across or down. To make this exercise more difficult do not look at the "Starters" paragraph below. It contains clues to the correct words to make from all the anagrams. The upside-down "Hint" at the very bottom of this page gives the correct answer to one of the anagram words.

1. **BELOW**   3. **ABIES**

2. **SHALE**   4. **ROSIE**

5. **HEWER**

Starters: These clues may help find the correct word hidden in each numbered anagram above: 1. Push aside. 2. Restraining device. 3. A count by his last name. 4. Willow 5. What place.

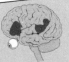

BRAIN BITES

Language is in many ways an invaluable aid to thought and memory. But Harvard memory researcher Daniel Schacter points out the flip side of that coin: "Verbally describing a face, a color, or even a taste of wine can impair subsequent recognition when an imprecise value description overrides a more precise nonverbal memory."

HINT: 4 = OSIER.

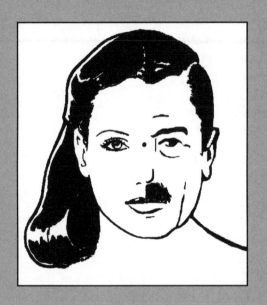

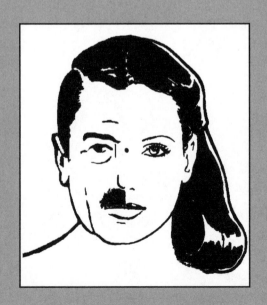

PUT ON YOUR HAPPY FACE

Face recognition is one of a number of kinds of "holistic" visual ability shown to be in the right hemisphere's domain of expertise. People with damage toward the rear of their right brain, in the occipital and temporal lobes, may have difficulty learning new faces, recognizing familiar faces, or even identifying a face as male or female.

The two faces on the opposite page are *chimeras*, meaning that they are composed of two half-faces joined together. Most people, if they focus on the dot in the center of each face in turn, find one to be more "female" than the other, even though they are exact mirror images. Since your left visual field (everything you see on the left side of the person's face if you're looking at his or her nose) connects to your right brain, which of the two chimeric faces would you *expect* to judge as more female, and which as more male — assuming your right brain dominates for facial processing?

B R A I N   B I T E S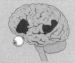

In our brains, the perception of emotion in the voice or face of another person is handled differently from feeling or expression of one's *own* emotion. Emotion researchers such as Drevets and Damasio have shown that the right hemisphere is specialized for the experience of only *negative* emotions, while the left handles *positive* emotions. One result of this is that left-brain stroke patients are more likely to be depressed than right-brain patients.

Thou must learn the alphabet, to wit, the order of the letters as they stand, perfectly without the book, and where every letter standeth: as (B) near the beginning, (N) about the middest, and (T) toward the end.

— Robert Cawdrey, *Table Alphabetical,* 1604

What a stupid thing is an old man learning an alphabet.

— Michel de Montaigne, *Essays,* II. 1580

ALPHABETICS

6 Letter-Elimination
Alphabet Interlocks
Self-Test: *Forbidden Words*

All about

ALPHABETICS

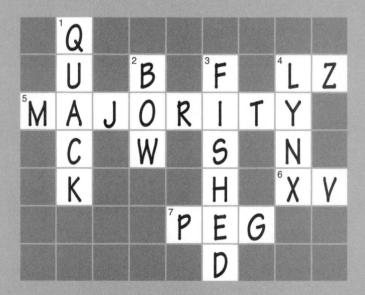

Alphabetics are crossword puzzles in which you use all 26 letters in the alphabet, but each letter only once. The process of elimination helps solve these puzzles more easily than most standard crosswords (though Alphabetics are not easier to construct). If you have solved most of the easy clues you have only a few letters left for the remaining difficult clues. Rearranging them, as you would in an anagram puzzle, helps you find the words that match the clues to fill the remaining spaces.

Though these exercises appear simple, they stimulate many parts of your brain, primarily the left hemisphere's ability to think of (or say) a word that matches the meaning given in a clue. *Aphasia*, the loss of some part of language ability, is suffered by about 40% of all stroke victims (especially right-handed men, whose language skills tend to be more isolated in the left brain than women's are).

The illustration on the next page includes the locations in the left brain of two major language-skill regions, both first discovered only about 130 years ago. Wernicke, a young German doctor, identified an area involved in understanding the meaning of words. Wernicke's aphasics speak fluently except that the words they use don't make sense — in severe cases, they speak nothing but "word salad." Some develop *paraphasia*, a tendency to paraphrase a word they just can't think of. Some can describe a situation but with tortured work-arounds because they cannot recall nouns (*anomia*). The sometimes-embarrassing, "tip-of-the-tongue" experience all normal people occasionally suffer tends to be caused by self-consciousness or emotional distraction or a temporary "overwriting" by a similar but more recent event

A few years before Wernicke's discovery, a French physician,

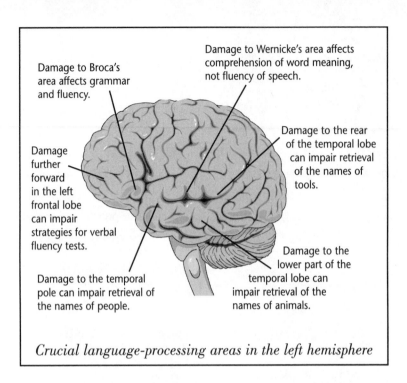

Damage to Broca's area affects grammar and fluency.

Damage to Wernicke's area affects comprehension of word meaning, not fluency of speech.

Damage to the rear of the temporal lobe can impair retrieval of the names of tools.

Damage further forward in the left frontal lobe can impair strategies for verbal fluency tests.

Damage to the temporal pole can impair retrieval of the names of people.

Damage to the lower part of the temporal lobe can impair retrieval of the names of animals.

Crucial language-processing areas in the left hemisphere

Paul Broca, treated a patient who could speak only the word "tan." When he died soon after, his brain showed damage in the part called the left frontal lobe. The type of aphasia that interferes with a patient's ability to recall how a word is spoken aloud, even though its meaning is perfectly clear, is called "Broca's aphasia." Tests of verbal fluency identify damage around Broca's area, as well as to temporal regions closer to Wernicke's area. In fact, damage to specific sites may cause problems retrieving the names for discrete categories of nouns: only animals or only tools, for example. The words for those things may not be "housed" in those specific spots, but those regions probably play an intermediate role in *accessing* them. Current electronic scanning technology can now pinpoint exactly where in the brain specific language skills are processed. For example, tests such as the part of the Wechsler battery that asks subjects to supply definitions for words (ranging from easy words like *winter* or *keen*, to harder ones such as *travesty* or *prolix*) cause areas in the left temporal lobe to light up, but not necessarily the same regions that light up when they're asked to supply categories of nouns such as the names of fruits or tools.

Some of the skills you'll be using to solve the following Alphabetics exercises are the same ones you need to do well on open-ended "fluency" tests that psychiatrists and neurologists use to assess possible brain damage. Those tests require the patient to list, in a minute, as many items as possible that fit a given category. For example, try to name as many mammals as you can in 60 seconds. Alternatively, try to list all the words you can that begin with the same letter or the same sound, *s*, for example. If you can correctly name 16-20 in 60 seconds, with no repeats, you are doing well; fewer than ten shows poor performance. Such tests show how well you can *access* the words in your mental lexicon, not how big a vocabulary you have. High word skills correlate with both age and education. Command of words will tend to rise at least until the middle years (the 50s or 60s) and begin a slow decline thereafter.

Occasionally, poor performance on verbal fluency tests can be caused by damage to the very front part of the left hemisphere, further forward than Broca's area. Why? The frontal lobes are generally involved in what are called "executive" functions — devising a strategy for achieving a goal, for example. When everything's working well in your brain, these strategies may be so automatic that you aren't even aware of them. If you were asked to name as many animals as you can, chances are you'd come up with a bigger list if you proceeded through the alphabet letter by letter, naming animals that begin with each letter in turn (aardvark, baboon, chinchilla, etc.) or break the larger category into smaller ones (pets, farm animals, etc.).

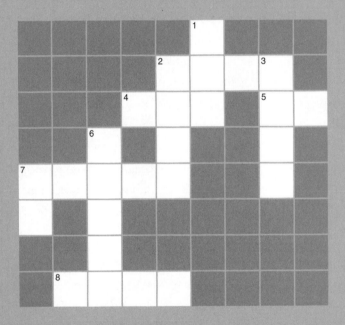

In this crossword puzzle format you will use each letter of the alphabet only once.

Across
2. Either side of a door opening
4. Not a lot
5. Frank Baum country
7. Rapid
8. Charon's waterway

Down
1. Ferret's foot
2. Sudden start
3. James name that was often his word
6. "_____-Horse Harry" Lee
7. Which see (Lat.)

Starters: 4 and 7 Across and 6 Down are good starting points.

BRAIN BITES

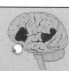

If you're a left-hander, how can you tell which of your brain hemispheres controls language? Jerre Levy and MaryLou Reid have proposed a simple test. If you write with your hand below the line of writing, as right-handers do, then your "language" hemisphere is opposite from your writing hand. If you write with your hand in a hooked position, then your left brain is dominant for controlling language, as it is for most right-handers. Some visual field tests support this theory.

HINT: 2 Across = jamb.

ALPHABETICS 2

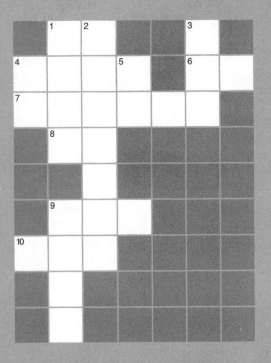

In this crossword puzzle format you will use each letter of the alphabet only once.

Across
1. Game board area (abbr.)
4. Plat du _____
6. 3-30 Mc., e.g.
7. Gaudy; flashy (slang)
8. AC opp.
9. Annoy
10. Public proclamation; prohibit

Down
1. Bought's partner
2. Stimulate
3. What for?
4. Navy Lt.'s ranking
5. Football lineman (abbr.)
9. Unscrupulous flirt

Starters: Use of an abbreviation in a clue signals that the solution is also abbreviated. 8, 9, and 10 Across and 1 and 5 Down are good starting points. 6 Across is the opposite of LF.

BRAIN BITES

If you go through the alphabet silently in your head, how many of the letters rhyme with "bee"? Next, how many letters, when printed as capitals, contain curves? Which task is easier for you? Researchers M. Coltheart, E. Hull, and D. Slater found that men were quicker and more accurate at the latter task, women quicker and more accurate at the former. This supports the generalization that women tend to be better at verbal skills, while men tend to be better at spatial skills.

HINT: 7 Across = glitzy.

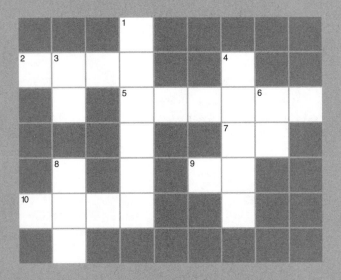

In this crossword puzzle format you will use each letter of the alphabet only once.

Across

2. Punch or dust, viz.
5. Harm; damage
7. TV spot
9. Entertainment host
10. Sleeveless garment

Down

1. Pledge; pickle
3. The yoke's on him
4. Charlatan
6. Address abbreviation
8. Turkish topper

Starters: 3 Down and 5 Across are good starting points.

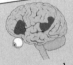

BRAIN BITES

For over one hundred years, it has been widely accepted that most people have strong left-hemisphere specialization for language. Recent research indicates that this may in fact be far more true for men than for women. In a reanalysis of older case studies of patients with brain damage, James Inglis and J. S. Lawson found that women were far less likely than men to suffer verbal or spatial deficits from damage to their left or right hemisphere. This would make sense if women's verbal and spatial centers are more evenly distributed across the two halves of their brain.

HINT: 1 Down = plight.

ALPHABETICS 4

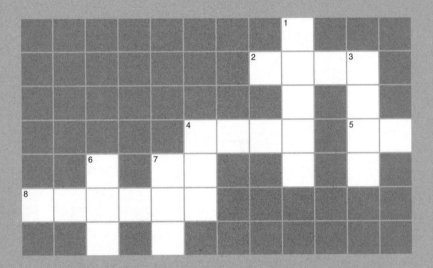

In this crossword puzzle format you will use each letter of the alphabet only once.

Across

2. Kind of button
4. Political coalition
5. Arboricultural degree
7. Dinner choice
8. Herbivore scraped its chin?

Down

1. Swift; hasty
3. Song of praise
4. Skivvies brand
6. Gab; yackety yak
7. Cowboy handle

Starters: 1 Down is a good starting point.

BRAIN BITES

Even though we often loosely say that the left hemisphere is "verbal" and the right "visual," these categories may not really reflect the brain's actual hemispheric division of labor. For example, neuropsychologist Elkhonon Goldberg points out that familiar symbols or icons, such as a letter of the alphabet or the circle with a line through it representing "no," are automatically processed by the left brain. Other less familiar visual images, such as a drawing of an irregular shape or an unfamiliar face, are handled more on the right side.

HINT: 5 Across = MF.

Alphabetics   53

ALPHABETICS 5

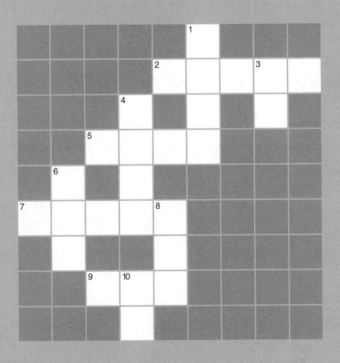

54

In this crossword puzzle format you will use each letter of the alphabet only once.

Across
2. Bee project
5. Pillage; plunder
7. Two-wheeled hybrid
9. Small fry interrogative

Down
1. Worthless stuff
3. He-man size probably (abbr.)
4. Daunt
6. Office at the Bijou
8. Prohibitionist
10. Powerful electrical abbreviation

Starters: 1 Down is a good starting point.

BRAIN BITES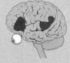

Many brain scientists have wondered whether it's just a coincidence that the left hemisphere controls both language and handedness. Canadian gender-and-brain researcher Doreen Kimura proposes that the link lies in the left hemisphere's control of fine motor movements. As the left hemisphere evolved to control motor skills in the hand (and perhaps to handle gestural communication), many of the same brain regions could have been recruited to manipulate the muscles required for speech.

HINT: 8 Down = dry.

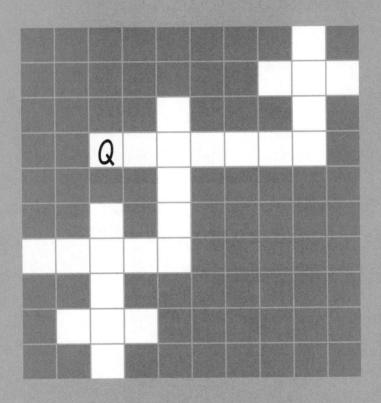

In this Alphabetics variant you will use each letter of the alphabet only once. What makes it different from the other puzzles in this category is that there are no clues to help you figure out which words to fill in. There are, of course, many possible solutions, but we have placed one letter in a box so your solution will be more likely to match ours. See the "Starters" section if you're stumped.

Starters: Move quickly if you're doing this at night. It will be good sport if you don't get boxed in.

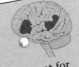

BRAIN BITES

Most humans are at least somewhat left-brain-dominant for speech. Most also have dominant control of fine motor skills in their left hemisphere, making them right-handed. Among humans living today in a cross-section of cultures, the incidence of right-handedness is about 90%. How long have we been this way? For many thousands of years, according to those, such as paleontologist Raymond Dart, who have analyzed cave paintings and stone tools dating from prehistoric times.

HINT: In our solution, two words that intersect with quickly are night and wavy.

WORD TO GUESS:	TABOO WORDS:
ant	*little, small, insect, grasshopper, termite*
wrench	*tool, nut, bolt, screw, turn*
vampire	*blood, fangs, bat, suck, Dracula*
chandelier	*light, candle, crystal, lamp, ceiling*
volcano	*mountain, lava, fire, erupt, hot*
ladder	*climb, fire, rungs, tree, building*
hyena	*Africa, scavenger, lion, predator, laugh*

WORD TO GUESS:	TABOO WORDS:
teardrop	*water, eye, cry, sad, wet*
curtain	*fabric, window, cloth, pull, draw*
brick	*wall, mortar, build, pig, cement*
cork	*bottle, stop, bark, wine, champagne*
mirror	*reflect, look, glass, break, luck*
parrot	*parakeet, bird, talk, polly, cracker*
soufflé	*air, egg, rise, light, puff*

FORBIDDEN WORDS

The part of your left frontal lobe around Broca's area is important for accessing the correct names for objects. So is a region
further back, near where the left temporal, parietal, and occipital lobes meet, known as the *angular gyrus*. Damage to this
region can result in *anomia*, or usually normal spontaneous
speech combined with the inability to think of the proper
names for objects on command. A related left-hemisphere
problem, *semantic paraphasia*, results in the need to provide
roundabout re-wordings of familiar objects (such as "red fruit"
for "tomato").

In this game (which requires at least one other player), you put
yourself in the role of someone who has to convey to someone
else what object you have in mind — only you're not allowed to
mention the object by name, nor are you permitted to use any
of five "taboo" words in your description. In effect, you're forc-
ing on yourself the kind of circumlocution some people have to
resort to because of brain damage. It's a real challenge. You
have two minutes total for all seven words on the list, then give
the book to your playing partner, and reverse roles with the
upside-down list.

Note: If a word is taboo, so is any word containing it (e.g.,
"sun" and "sunburn").

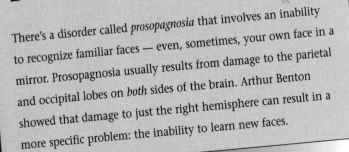

BRAIN BITES

There's a disorder called *prosopagnosia* that involves an inability
to recognize familiar faces — even, sometimes, your own face in a
mirror. Prosopagnosia usually results from damage to the parietal
and occipital lobes on *both* sides of the brain. Arthur Benton
showed that damage to just the right hemisphere can result in a
more specific problem: the inability to learn new faces.

*Interdependence   absolute,   forseen,
ordained, decreed*

— Rudyard Kipling, *M'Andrew's Hymn,* 1893

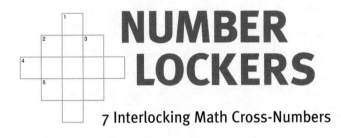

NUMBER
LOCKERS

7 Interlocking Math Cross-Numbers

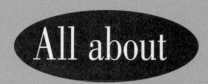

All about

NUMBER LOCKERS

1	**2**		**3**	**4**
	5	**6**		
		7		
8	**9**			
10			**11**	

N umber lockers are a kind of crossword puzzle with the clues leading you to numbers rather than words. In the answers, you're allowed to use any whole numbers from 1 to 9; fractions, negative numbers, and 0 aren't allowed.

To solve Number lockers, you don't need to know anything beyond the most basic algebra, but you might want to refresh your memory about the meaning of a few terms. A *square* is a number derived by multiplying a number by itself; for example, 9 is the square of 3 (3 x 3 = 9). If you multiply a number by itself twice, you get a *cube*; 27 is the cube of 3 (3 x 3 x 3 = 27). A *square* (or *cube*) *root* is the number that, when multiplied by itself, yields the square (or cube); for example, 3 is the square root of 9, and the cube root of 27. Above cube, we'll use the term *power*: 16 is 2 to the fourth power (2 x 2 x 2 x 2 = 16).

Most numbers aren't squares or cubes of any whole number. 16 is a square (of 4). 18 is not (of any whole number). 8 is a cube (of 2), but not a square. 9 is a square (of 3), but not a cube. If a clue asks you for a cube that fits a single-digit space, you know it must be either 1 or 8 (1 x 1 x 1 = 1; 2 x 2 x 2 = 8). If we ask you for a cube that fits 2 spaces, the answer could be 27 (3 x 3 x 3) or 64 (4 x 4 x 4). Any other cube would be too short (the cube of 1 or 2, either of which would be a single-digit number) or too long (the cube of 5 or higher, which would be a triple-or-more-digit number; for example, 5 x 5 x 5 = 125).

A *prime number* can be divided only by itself and 1 without leaving a remainder. 3 is a prime number; so are 5, 7, 11, 13, etc. 21 is not a prime number because it can also be divided by 3 and by 7. *1 is not a prime number.*

Consecutive numbers are numbers that follow one another in a sequence, like counting consecutively from a lower to a higher number. (In the rare clues asking for descending consecutive numbers, the clue or hint will say "descending.") Example: "consecutive odd digits" can be the sequence 1, 3, 5, 7, 9, in that order. (When *five* boxes must be filled by that clue, those can be the *only* possible answers since you can use only single-digit numbers.)

Smallest or *largest possible number* means that the answer cannot have more or fewer digits than the number of boxes available for that clue. For example, the smallest possible square of a prime number that will fit in a two-digit answer is 25 (5 x 5).

Another important word to remember is *palindrome*. A palindrome (literally "running back" in Greek) is any phrase, word, or number that reads the same backwards and forwards. The phrase referring to the Emperor Napoleon's exile, "Able was I ere I saw Elba," is a palindrome, as is the word "redder." A palindromic number might be 33, or 787, etc.

Unities are ones (11 or 111, etc.). So "a cube of unities" that must fit into four boxes *must* be the cube of 11, which is 1331.

A *product* of a number is the result of multiplying that number by any other number. For example, a product of 15 is 45 (15 x 3); so is 60, and 150.

As with crosswords, you can start with easy clues and use those answers to help you solve more difficult intersecting ones. If you take a look at the clues in the example at the top of the opposite page, you can see that there are many possible answers for 1 Across, so that wouldn't be a good "entry" for this puzzle.

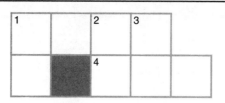

Across
1. A palindrome
4. A palindrome in which the first digit is the square root of the last two

Down
1. Odd number to the fourth power
2. A square
3. Digits add up to 10

However, if you look at 1 Down, "Odd number to the fourth power," there's only one possible answer. A moment's trial-and-error calculation will show you that there are only two fourth-power numbers with two digits: 16 (2 x 2 x 2 x 2) and 81 (3 x 3 x 3 x 3). Only the second option could be correct here because the clue states that you need an *odd* number.

Once you get 1 Down, you also know the last digit in 1 Across (since 1 Across is a palindrome), and you therefore also know 3 Down.

What about 2 Down? There are several possible answers, but only one of them (25) lets you get an answer that fits the clue to the intersecting 4 Across. Finally, the fact that 1 Across is a palindrome lets you fill in the final digit there:

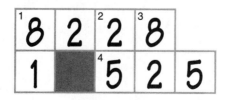

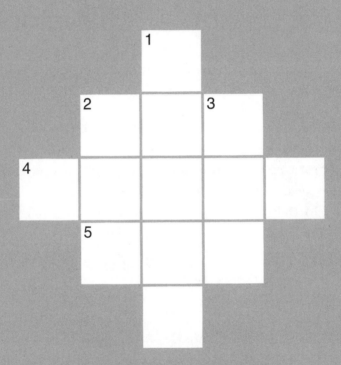

Across

2. A palindrome that is the cube of a prime number which is in turn a single digit
4. Palindrome that begins with 5
5. A dozen's dozen

Down

1. Two unities to the fourth power, and a palindrome at that
2. Two digits descent to 1, one at a time
3. This adds up to 9

Starters: Remember, *palindromes* are numbers that read the same backwards and forwards.

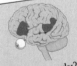

BRAIN BITES

Can you raise your SAT scores by keeping a tennis ball handy? Canadian psychologist Bernard Schiff has reported that you can stimulate the activity of one brain hemisphere, affecting your emotions and perhaps switching on that hemisphere's distinctive problem-solving abilities, by squeezing a tennis ball with the opposite hand. So if you want to solve word or number problems, try squeezing the ball with your right hand (stimulating the left brain).

HINT: 1 Down is 14641.

Across

2. The second digit is the cube of the first
3. The lowest possible three-digit square of an even number (Remember, no zeros allowed)
4. The cube of the number that made the square in 3 Across
5. The sum of the digits is 22

Down

1. A palindrome: the first or third digit is half the second
2. Each digit is half the corresponding first four digits in 1 Down
3. The sum of the digits is 13
4. Both square and fourth power of even numbers

Starters: Remember, *palindromes* are numbers that read the same backwards and forwards. A *square* is a number produced by multiplying another, smaller number by itself. To produce a *cube*, multiply a number by itself and then again by that product (e.g., the cube of 3 is 27: 3 x 3 x 3 = 27).

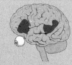

B R A I N   B I T E S

Language skills can be an aid to arithmetic calculation because language provides labels for numbers and mathematical operations. But language and computational abilities don't reduce to a single skill housed in the same area of the brain. Medical researchers Stanislaus Dehaene and Lauren Cohen have studied brain-damaged patients who can count but not calculate, and others who can calculate but not name the numbers or operations involved.

HINT: 2 Down is 2424.

NUMBER LOCKER 3

	1	2	3	
4				5
6			7	
8		9		
	10			

Across

1. The second and third digits are the square of the first, which is itself a cube (even number)
4. The first digit is the same as the last (even number)
6. Prime number
7. The sum of the digits is 11 (even number)
8. The sum of the digits is 24 (odd number)
10. Odd number whose digits increase by threes

Down

1. The first two digits are the square and the last three are the cube of a number which is itself a square (odd number)
2. Even number which is both a square and a cube
3. The first two digits are the square of a prime number, the last three the cube of the same prime number
4. The cube of an even number; the sum of its digits is 9
5. The square of 6 Across; the sum of its digits is 19
9. Square of the number found in 4 Down; the sum of its digits is 9

Starters: A good "entry" for this puzzle is 1 Across. Given the information that 1 Across starts with a one-digit cube, and that the second and third are that first digit's square, there's only one possible answer; then, it's easy to get 1, 2, and 3 Down. Remember, a *prime number* is divisible only by itself and 1.

HINT: 4 Across is 21492.

Number Locker 4

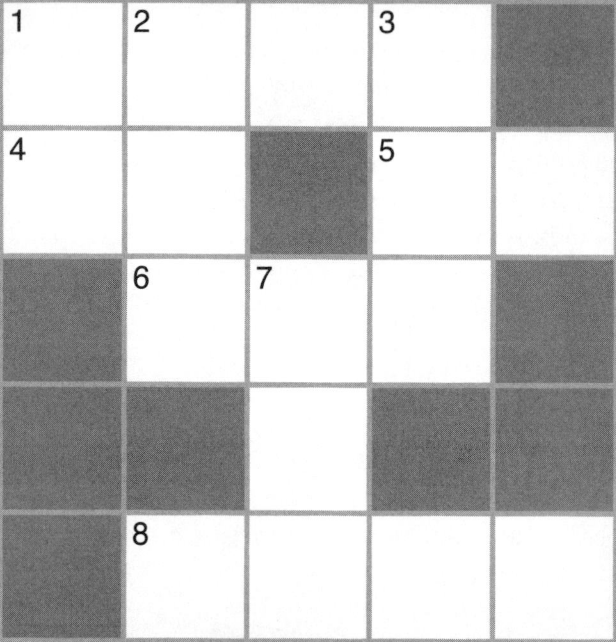

Across

1. The cube of a prime number (palindrome)
4. The square of a cube
5. The cube of a digit in 1 Across
6. Descending consecutive numbers
8. Square a square; now you square that

Down

1. The square of a square
2. The cube of a prime number (palindrome)
3. The square of a prime number (palindrome)
7. In reverse, the cube of a cube (odd number)

Starters: There's only one possible answer for 4 Across

BRAIN BITES

San Jose State University professor Irene T. Miura points out that Japanese children tend to learn the numbers between 10 and 100 at a younger age than their English-speaking counterparts, because Japanese number-words are more transparently composed of the names for numbers 1 through 9. (*Zyuuni* "twelve," for example, is literally *zyuu* "ten" plus *ni* "two" — "ten-two.") This helps them learn the concepts of addition, too.

HINT: The answer to 7
Down is 215.

Number Lockers 73

Number Locker 5

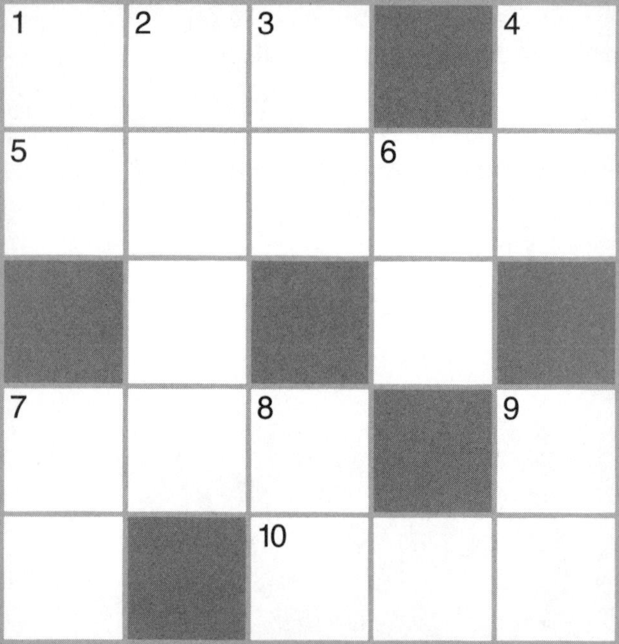

Across

1. The cube of a prime number: first and third digits are the same
5. Count a palindrome by threes
7. Another palindrome with threes
10. A gross number

Down

1. A square; see 6 and 7 Down
2. Digits descend one at a time
3. The second number is the square of the first
4. Un-square route
6. See 1 Down
7. See 6 Down
8. Its sum is one-third of the square root of 10 Across
9. Sunny Louis

Starters: A good "entry" for this puzzle is 3 Down; of the two possible answers, you can exclude one by looking at 1 Across.

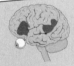

BRAIN BITES

Those people who cluster at the extreme high end of math scores tend to be men. The reasons aren't all cultural. Men from all cultures tend to perform better than women at mental rotations of 3-dimensional objects. Some babies are born with the correct chromosomal makeup of a male — an X and a Y chromosome — but lack receptors for male hormones such as testosterone. (As infants they even look enough like girls to fool a doctor.) Later in school, they tend to have lower math scores than normal boys.

HINT: 5 Across is 63936.

NUMBER LOCKER 6

Across

1. These even numbers add up to 16; the first and last numbers are the same
4. An even number
5. Square of 1 Down
6. The first digit is three less than the second (even number)
8. Palindromic 19th-century date

Down

1. Square of a prime number
2. The first two digits are the same as the last two (even number)
3. Square of an odd number; multiple of 1 Down
5. The sum of the digits is 8
7. Square of an odd number

Starters: A good "entry" for this puzzle is 1 Down; of the two possible answers, you can exclude one by looking at 3 Down, given the stipulation in 1 Across.

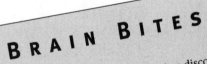

BRAIN BITES

Brain researcher Steven Gaulin has discovered that in bird and mammal species in which the males are polygamous (one male mates with as many females as he can, instead of settling down with just one), those polygamous males tend to have better maze-running abilities and a larger hippocampus — a locus in the brain of spatial intelligence. So human males' somewhat superior math and spatial skills and their notorious sexual promiscuity may both have a single biological cause.

Hint: 2 Down is 482248.

NUMBER LOCKER 7

Across

1. One-half of 3 Across
3. Square of an even number
5. The digits are all odd; each one is greater than the one before
7. The square of the sum of the first two digits in 4 Down
8. The digits are alternatingly even and odd; each is greater than the one before
10. Square of a prime number
11. A number that's the same upside-down

Down

2. Square of a number that is itself a square
3. An odd number; the fifth digit is the square of the first; the middle three digits are the cube of the fifth
4. The sum of the first two digits is the sum of the third (odd number)
6. Together, the first two digits are a multiple of the third (even number)
8. The next even square after 3 Across
9. The first digit is the square root of 10 Across

Starters: A good "entry" for this puzzle is 10 Across, along with 8 Down and 3 Across. (Each has two to three possible answers, but together only answer one is possible for each.)

BRAIN BITES

As men age, their hippocampus — a structure in the brain linked to math and spatial skills — shrinks more rapidly than in women, and testosterone levels drop. Biological changes such as these may help explain why mathematicians (who tend to be men) peak at such a young age.

Hint: 3 Down is 37299.

Man is so made that when anything fires his soul impossibilities vanish.

— Jean de la Fontaine, *Fables,* VOL. VIII, 1671

You write, "it is impossible": *that is not French.*

— Napoleon I, *Letter to Count Lemarois,* July 9, 1813

POSSIBLE PAIRS

4 Concept-Correlations
(for 2 people)
Self-Test: *Proverbial Pairs*

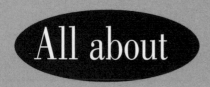

All about

POSSIBLE PAIRS

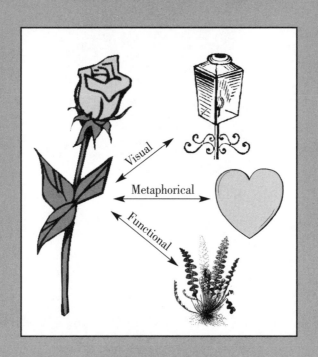

P ossible Pairs puzzles are ones that can be solved either by a "right-brain" or a "left-brain" approach. The puzzles challenge you to group a collection of objects into pairs, by whatever rules you choose. There's no right answer, and no preordained level of difficulty. (Psychologists sometimes refer to this kind of test as a "divergent production" task, as opposed to the "convergent," single-right-answer questions you get on a typical IQ test.) It's fun to do these puzzles with a partner, each of you working independently and then seeing if your answers agree. Your partner's matching rationale might be completely different from your own.

Functional matches are left-brain, visual or metaphorical matches are right-brain. If one of you pairs up images that share an important function, tools for example, that person's left hemisphere has taken over the job. But when a person links objects because they are the same shape or share a metaphorical connection or punning double meaning, the right brain is more likely to be doing the work.

These puzzles give you insight into how language works because categorization — grouping things into classes and attaching labels to those classes — is also a fundamental part of language. Picture-matching tests given to brain-damaged patients show that the left brain is more likely to match objects according to functional attributes (a knife and a loaf of bread, for example), while the right brain matches by visual similarity (a knife and a ruler, say).

Ever since Paul Broca, it's been accepted that (in his words) "we speak with the left hemisphere." More recent research has refined Broca's views. About 95% of right-handed men have a left hemisphere that's dominant for the most uniquely human aspects of communication, those aspects linguists refer to as *syntax* (sentence structure) and *semantics* (meaning). Recent studies using state-of-the-art neuroimaging technology have revealed that women are less strongly *lateralized* for language than men — they tend to use both sides of their brain more than men do. People who are left-handed or with mixed handedness also tend to have language centers more evenly distributed across the two halves of the brain. (That explains why right-handed men are slower to recover their language abilities after a left-hemisphere stroke.)

Some other aspects of communication (including what linguists call *pragmatics*) are less clearly left-brain-centered even for right-handed men. The right hemisphere plays a role in controlling prosody (vocal intonation) and manual gestures. Humor and "indirect" discourse — figuring out what people mean when they say, "Gee, I'd sure like some help washing these dishes" — can also be affected by right-brain damage. Some people with right-brain damage have a difficult time interpreting indirect requests, and some researchers have concluded that the right hemisphere plays a role in drawing *inferences* from conversation. In the example above, the request to help with the dishes is an inference you might draw even though it's not literally expressed in the words. By a process of elimination, the left hemisphere is more literal-minded.

Recent work with PET scans confirms that metaphorical language — describing investors as squirrels gathering nuts for the winter, say, or understanding the word *green* to mean "inexperienced" — is also processed partly in the right brain. Some such studies support the theory that it's the right brain that plays a role in quickly activating many possible senses of a word or phrase, including figurative ones, and the left brain that selects just one and suppresses the others; the left brain on its own is less able to generate the broad range of senses to begin with.

To get an idea how the right hemisphere plays a crucial role in humor, consider the story about Niels Bohr, the Nobel Prize-winning physicist. A visitor to Bohr's office, noticing a good-luck horseshoe hung above the door, exclaimed, "Surely *you* don't believe in that superstitious nonsense, Doctor Bohr!" Bohr's reply: "Of course not, but I've heard it works whether you believe in it or not."

Jokes like this are hard to explain to somebody who doesn't "get" them — which is itself a clue that the relatively nonverbal right hemisphere is doing a lot of the work necessary to detect the humor. The best we can do is something like this. The humor lies in the juxtaposition of multiple contradictory things: Bohr's rational disbelief in the good-luck power of a horseshoe, and his apparent belief that it may have such power after all, mediated by a sober pragmatism that lets him have it both ways. The right brain has no problem holding multiple contradictory notions in its mind at once. The left brain must pick out just one notion, and discard the contradictions. This joke also serves as a nice illustration of the right brain's contribution because the very symbolism of the horseshoe — its role as a good-luck metaphor — is something the literal-minded left brain might miss altogether.

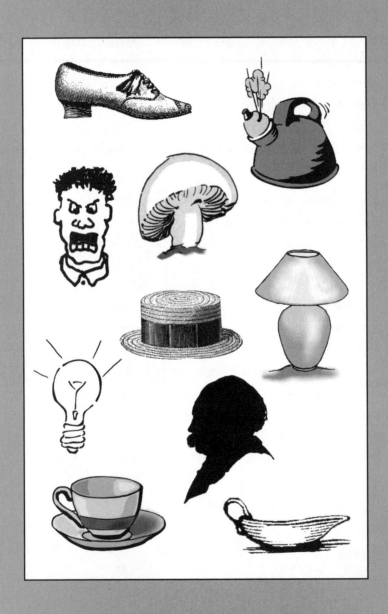

Make five pairs out of these 10 different items. Use each picture once and don't leave any pictures out. Pair them so that all five are the *best* combinations, based on whatever similarities make most sense to you. There is no "correct" solution; some possibilities are given on the answer page.

For fun, try this one with a friend, and see if you both match the items in the same way. Score two points for each pair of yours that matches your friend's answer, and zero points for each pair that doesn't match. Eight to 10 points: like minds. Four to six points: keep talking. Zero to two points: different planets.

BRAIN BITES

Not all language abilities are housed in the left hemisphere, even in the typical right-handed man. Intelligence researchers Howard Gardner and Ellen Winner found that people whose brain is damaged on the right side have difficulty understanding metaphor or getting the punchline of a joke.

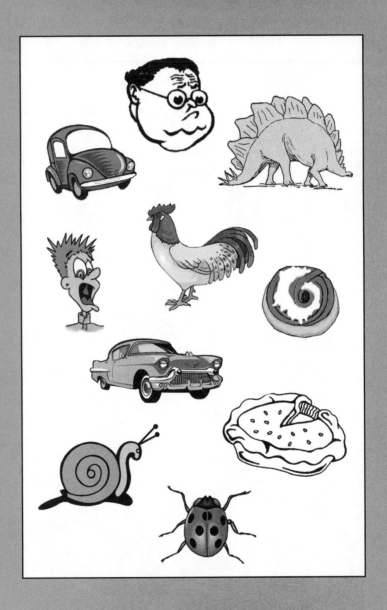

Make five pairs out of these 10 different items. Use each picture once and don't leave any pictures out. Pair them so that all five are the *best* combinations, based on whatever similarities make most sense to you. There is no "correct" solution; some possibilities are given on the answer page.

For fun, try this one with a friend, and see if you both match the items in the same way. Score two points for each pair of yours that matches your friend's answer, and zero points for each pair that doesn't match. Eight to 10 points: like minds. Four to six points: keep talking. Zero to two points: different planets.

BRAIN BITES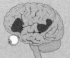

In a recent functional magnetic resonance imaging (fMRI) study of blood flow in the brains of men and women performing a rhyming task, researchers Bennett and Sally Shaywitz and colleagues found evidence for strong sex differences in brain activity. For all 19 men in the study, the fMRI revealed blood flow in an area of the left frontal lobe. Eight of the women also showed more left-side activity, although less strongly asymmetrical, while 11 of the women showed blood flow evenly on both sides of their brain. This supports other research findings that show less left-hemisphere specialization for language among women than among men.

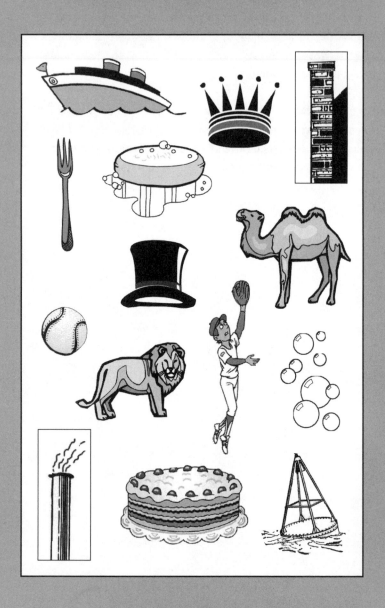

Make seven pairs out of these 14 different items. Use each picture once and don't leave any pictures out. Pair them so that all five are the *best* combinations, based on whatever similarities make most sense to you. There is no "correct" solution; some possibilities are given on the answer page.

For fun, try this one with a friend, and see if you both match the items in the same way. Score two points for each pair of yours that matches your friend's answer, and zero points for each pair that doesn't match. Twelve to 14 points: like minds. Eight to 10 points: keep talking. Zero to six points: different planets.

BRAIN BITES

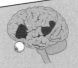

Some left-brain strokes are so specific in their effect that the patient will forget just one single class of words, such as the names for fruits or vegetables. In a recent PET scan study, University of Iowa brain researchers Hanna and Antonio Damasio identified three different regions of the left temporal lobe involved in naming three different word categories: names of people, animals, and tools. (The people-naming task also activated the right temporal lobe.) Since the "animals" region is between the other two, it's much more common for a brain lesion to result in a combined "people/animals" or "tools/animals" naming deficit than a combined "people/tools" deficit.

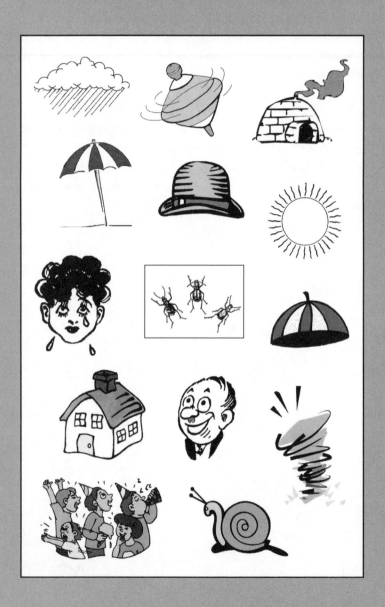

Make seven pairs out of these 14 different items. Use each picture once and don't leave any pictures out. Pair them so that all five are the *best* combinations, based on whatever similarities make most sense to you. There is no "correct" solution; some possibilities are given on the answer page.

For fun, try this one with a friend, and see if you both match the items in the same way. Score two points for each pair of yours that matches your friend's answer, and zero points for each pair that doesn't match. Twelve to 14 points: like minds. Eight to 10 points: keep talking. Zero to six points: different planets.

BRAIN BITES

Some EEG studies show that Multiple Personality Disorder results from shifts in dominance between the two hemispheres. Neuropsychologist Polly Henninger argues that, if there's one mature, well-adjusted personality, it relates to the left hemisphere, while the other, "alter," personalities are associated with the right. This fits psychiatrist Fredric Schiffer's "dual-brain" theory that productive/unproductive, mature/immature psychological conflicts in many of us might be attributed to shifts in dominant brain activity from one hemisphere to the other.

1. Absence makes the heart grow fonder.
2. Why buy a cow when milk is so cheap?
3. Children and fools tell the truth.
4. All things come to those who wait.
5. Where bees are, there is honey.
6. Look before you leap.
7. Opposites attract.
8. Don't change horses in mid-stream.
9. There's no such thing as a free lunch.
10. Don't throw good money after bad.
11. Honesty is the best policy.
12. The early bird gets the worm.
13. Hasty climbers have sudden falls.
14. Out of sight, out of mind.
15. He who hesitates is lost.
16. Don't cross the bridge until you come to it.
17. Make hay while the sun shines.
18. Throw dirt enough, and some will stick.
19. You can't judge a book by its cover.
20. The truth will out.
21. Two heads are better than one.
22. Birds of a feather flock together.
23. All that glitters is not gold.
24. Too many cooks spoil the broth.
25. You only get free cheese in a mousetrap.
26. The cowl does not make the monk.

PROVERBIAL PAIRS

Even though proverbs are supposed to capture important timeless truths, they can be hard to interpret in plain, everyday language. (Try *A rolling stone gathers no moss*, for example.) And
if proverbs are so true and timeless, why is it that you can find
so many contradictory ones?

Take a look at the sayings on the opposite page, and group
them together if they convey roughly the same thing in different ways ("synonymous proverbs"), *or* if they express conflict-
ing wisdom ("antonymous proverbs"). (Hint: not every proverb
will have an antonymous counterpart, not every one has a synonymous version, and some proverbs have multiple syn-
onyms.) For an added final challenge, see if you can come up
with a rationalization for the antonymous proverbs such that
both can still be viewed as valid.

This puzzle exercises both hemispheres' language centers,
since the right hemisphere has been shown to make an important contribution to the interpretation of proverbs and
metaphorical language in general. People with right-brain damage often have overly literal interpretations of proverbs that fail
to capture the essence of the proverb's meaning. So do schizo-
phrenics. (When asked to interpret *The bread never falls but on
its buttered side*, for example, they may explain that "the buttered side is heavier.") If you take the added step of providing
a rationalization for the antonymous proverbs' compatibility,
then you're relying on your left brain's "interpreter" mechanism, according to brain researcher Michael Gazzaniga.

There are no "right" or "wrong" answers. Our groupings are on
the answer page.

How forcible are right words!

— The Book of Job 6:25, circa 325 B.C.

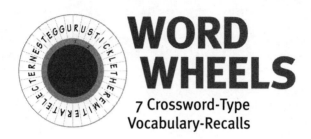

WORD WHEELS

7 Crossword-Type Vocabulary-Recalls

All about

WORD WHEELS

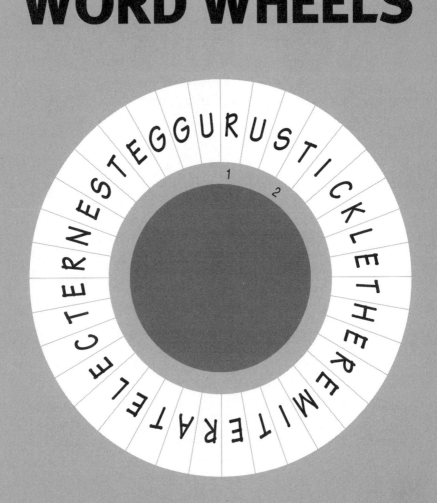

W ord Wheels tap the same regions of your brain that you use to solve crossword puzzles. In fact, Word Wheels are just like crossword puzzles except that *overlapping* words, rather than *intersecting* ones, help you to solve the clues.

If you take a look at the circle on the opposite page, you'll see what might at first seem like just a random assortment of letters arranged in a circle. But look a little more carefully, and you'll see that those letters actually form regular English words, as long as you draw divisions in the right places. Starting with the letter above the number 1 and working clockwise, you'll find the word *rustic* (or *rust*); at number 2, you'll find *tickle* (or *tick*), and so on. This Word Wheel could be the solution to a puzzle with "rural" as the first clue, and "amuse" as the second, etc. Since the answers always overlap one or more letters in the next word, each one helps you solve, or check your solutions for, the pre- ceding and following answers. Eventually, the words come back full circle as the final one (in this example, the answer to a clue such as "spiritual leader") joins up with the first. Unlike the Word Wheel on the facing page, all the other exercises in this chapter come equipped with numbers inserted at the beginning of each new word that correspond to numbered clues. However, we deleted the remaining numbers 3 to 15 from this Word Wheel so you could try to find the additional 13 overlapping words and insert the correct number below the first letter of each new word around the circle.

That's all there is to the rules of this game. But before you rush ahead to try your hand at solving the puzzles, here's some inter- esting information about the skills you'll be using. And yes, there *will* be a test afterwards. Some terms are used in the exercises that follow.

In the 18th century, people who studied the human brain believed that all of its parts did pretty much the same work. The dogma was that the two halves of the brain were simple mirror images of each other, and that the brain functioned as an undifferentiated unit, with no particular skill tied to any specific region.

By the 20th century, that received wisdom had changed, due mostly to 19th-century physicians who made careful observations that damage to different parts of their patients' brains caused different effects on their behavior. A young French surgeon named Paul Broca noted that many of his patients with speech problems were revealed, on autopsy, to have had *lesions* (injuries) in a certain area of the left frontal lobe. These patients had difficulty with "expressive" aspects of language, that is, with expressing themselves fluently and with the proper grammatical parts of speech and inflections (a condition known as *agrammatism*). The term now used for language disorders like this is *aphasia* (Broca himself used the word *aphemia*), literally meaning "no speech"; people who have speech dysfunctions caused by brain damage (from a stroke, for example) are called *aphasics*. The kind of "expressive" aphasia Broca described came to be called *Broca's aphasia*, and the region in the left frontal lobe he observed to be the site of the problem is called *Broca's area*.

Another pioneer in developing the doctrine of cerebral localization — the idea that different parts of the brain handle different functions — was a German neurologist named Karl Wernicke. Wernicke noted that lesions farther back from Broca's area, in the the left temporal lobe, often led to difficulty understanding the speech of others. These patients seemed fluent enough, but their own speech was meaningless, and they seemed unaware that they had a problem at all. This kind of "receptive" language problem came to be called *Wernicke's aphasia*, and the part of the brain involved is called *Wernicke's area*.

Since Broca and Wernicke's time, many refinements have been made in our understanding of the left hemisphere's language centers. Damage to regions other than Broca's or Wernicke's may produce different, sometimes very specific, problems. A lesion in the left frontal lobe can cause *avocalia* (also known as *amusia*), an inability to sing; an injury to a corresponding part of the right brain can impair musical pitch and rhythm. The left frontal region involved in avocalia isn't the same as Broca's area, since Broca's aphasics can sometimes sing quite fluently. Some therapists help Broca's aphasics re-learn language skills by teaching them to "sing" word sequences, and then gradually deemphasize the melody. Clinicians have been able to tease apart language and mathematical calculation abilities by observing different regions of the left hemisphere involved in the two. Some patients may have no language problem as such but difficulty calculating (*acalculia*), while others can calculate but can't name the resulting product. Damage to the *angular gyrus*, a region behind Wernicke's area, can result in *alexia* (inability to read) and *agraphia* (inability to write).

Because Broca's area is involved in the fluent retrieval of words that match the meaning you want to convey, and Wernicke's area is crucial for what linguists call *semantics*, or meaning, you'll be using both of these left-brain regions to solve these Word Wheel puzzles.

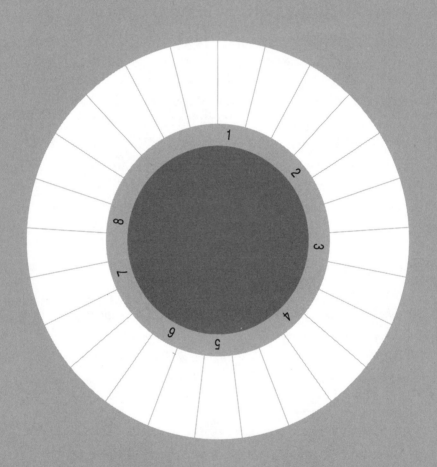

Just as one word leads to another, words lead into each other,
or overlap. If you start in slot #1 with the right word, you
should have little trouble completing the circle with 7 additional overlapping words. Each word starts in a numbered slot that
corresponds to the number of the clue.

Clues

1. Response
2. Brain research pioneer
   Karl _____
3. Buffalo Head
4. Temperature scale

5. Nice wine
6. Scandinavians of yore
7. Join with stitches
8. Memory loss

Starters: If you're stumped by #4, go to #5: #3 and #5 meet to
fill in the answer to #4.

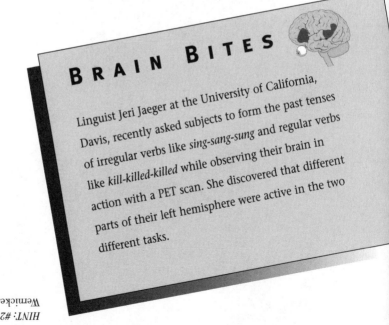

BRAIN BITES

Linguist Jeri Jaeger at the University of California,
Davis, recently asked subjects to form the past tenses
of irregular verbs like *sing-sang-sung* and regular verbs
like *kill-killed-killed* while observing their brain in
action with a PET scan. She discovered that different
parts of their left hemisphere were active in the two
different tasks.

*HINT: #2 is
Wernicke.*

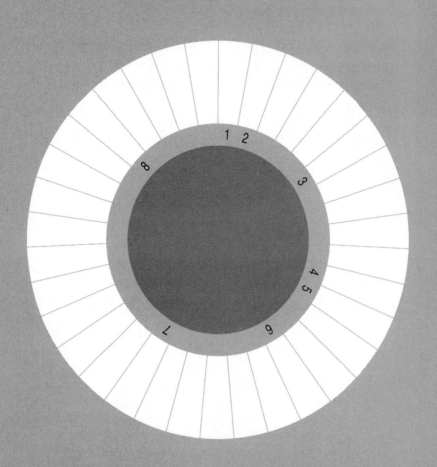

Just as one word leads to another, words lead into each other,
or overlap. If you start in slot #1 with the right word, you
should have little trouble completing the circle with 7 additional overlapping words. Each word starts in a numbered slot that
corresponds to the number of the clue.

Clues

1. Sound of a Bic
2. Played lightly over; thrashed
3. Send to school
4. Expressing end or purpose

5. Bring out
6. Court summons; Kentucky
   Derby winner
7. "Cuckoo" hence cuckoo, e.g.
8. Using certain poetic feet

Starters: #1 is Clack's brother.

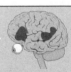

BRAIN BITES

Vocabulary-based language skills are one aspect of intelligence
that tends to improve with age. Some other aspects, especially
ones that require you to perform rapid calculations or filter out
extraneous details, tend to decline. But both kinds can be
improved or maintained with practice — by solving word and
number puzzles such as these, for example.

HINT: #1 is another example of #7; #4 is telic.

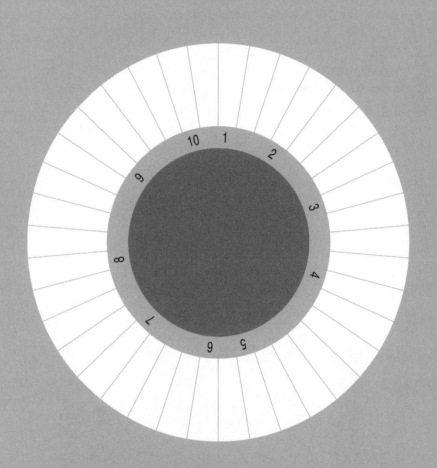

Just as one word leads to another, words lead into each other, or overlap. If you start in slot #1 with the right word, you should have little trouble completing the circle with 9 additional overlapping words. Each word starts in a numbered slot that corresponds to the number of the clue.

Clues

1. Collette wrote with one
2. Rubeola
3. Brain injury
4. New York neighbor
5. _____ up (admit)

6. Brain cell
7. Beginning
8. Teapot brouhaha
9. Mark of disgrace
10. Traveler's aid

Starters: #2 causes quarantines.

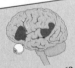

BRAIN BITES

Which of these two sentences is easier for you to understand? *The lion that the zookeeper let loose ate the dog*, or *The zookeeper let loose the lion that ate the dog?* For speakers of almost all languages, the kind of "center-embedded" structure in the first version is harder to process and is often avoided. In some languages, center-embedding is downright ungrammatical. A recent PET scan study by K. Stromswold and colleagues showed that center-embedded constructions result in increased blood flow to the brain's left frontal lobe, which they suggest might reveal a greater memory load imposed by such structures.

HINT: #9 is stigma.

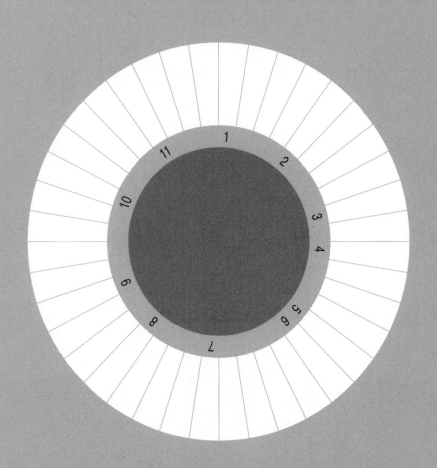

Just as one word leads to another, words lead into each other, or overlap. If you start in slot #1 with the right word, you should have little trouble completing the circle with 10 additional overlapping words. Each word starts in a numbered slot that corresponds to the number of the clue.

Clues

1. One who's lost the power of speech
2. Hammer's erstwhile Russian partner
3. For fear that
4. Common cause of brain damage
5. Knowledge; mental perception
6. Military banner
7. The left brain matches these to faces
8. Redundant hoosegow halved
9. One with *agrammatism* has trouble with this
10. Grecian Diana
11. Accident

Starters: The prefix *a-* in *agrammatism* means "not." The sequence of letters that immediately follows should help reveal the answer.

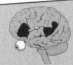

BRAIN BITES

Is it easier for you to tap rhythmically with the right or left hand while talking? For most people, it's easier with the left. The tasks that interfere with each other the least are likely to be controlled by opposite hemispheres. So if you're left-brain dominant for language, as most people are, right-handed tapping is controlled by that same side of the brain and confusion results.

HINT: *The Greek counterpart of Diana is Artemis.*

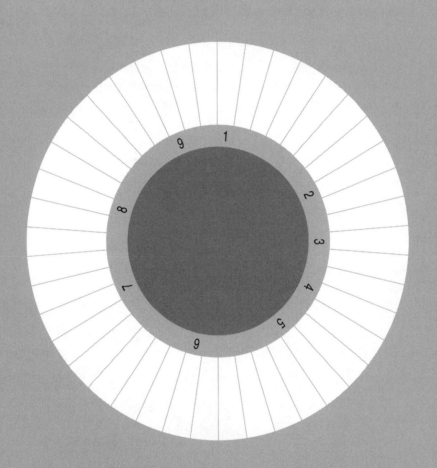

Just as one word leads to another, words lead into each other, or overlap. If you start in slot #1 with the right word, you should have little trouble completing the circle with 8 additional overlapping words. Each word starts in a numbered slot that corresponds to the number of the clue.

Clues

1. Symbolic picture, e.g.
2. Plant louse
3. Notion
4. Hymn of praise
5. Half a cerebrum

6. Nonconformist
7. What people with *acalculia* can't do
8. Quarterback's option
9. Like some excuses

Starters: #5 is also half of the terrestrial globe.

BRAIN BITES

Even though language relies heavily on left-brain skills, particular writing systems may tap the abilities of either hemisphere. Written Japanese uses two systems of symbols, *Kanji* and *Kana*. According to researchers Sasanuma and Fujimura, Japanese right-hemisphere stroke patients have a hard time with *Kanji*, Chinese-based ideographic symbols that encode an *image or idea* rather than sounds. However, patients with damage to their left hemisphere have a harder time with *Kana* because its symbols directly encode *sound* (specifically, syllables, as do the letters of the alphabet we use for English).

HINT: #6 is heretic.

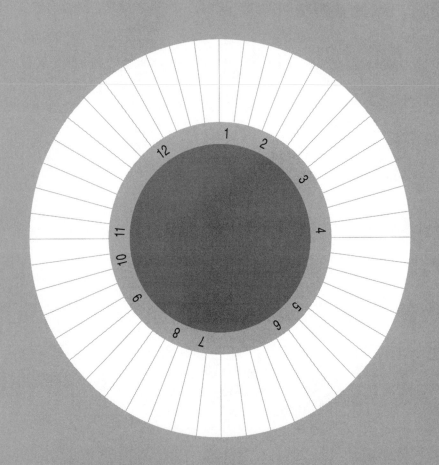

Just as one word leads to another, words lead into each other, or overlap. If you start in slot #1 with the right word, you should have little trouble completing the circle with 11 additional overlapping words. Each word starts in a numbered slot that corresponds to the number of the clue.

Clues

1. Deals with words
2. Ship stabilizer
3. Stellar adjective; star-shaped
4. Soup that's a real character builder
5. Navigational abbr.
6. Do not _____!

7. Fruit-bearing tree
8. Descendant
9. New and different
10. Eliminate; shorten
11. Inscribed symbol perhaps
12. Substantial; imposing

Starters: #5 is not ETA. *War and Peace* once was and still is an example of #9.

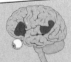

BRAIN BITES

Drawing on psychologists Postman and Underwood's concept of *interference*, memory researcher Daniel Schacter suggests a harmless reason for apparent memory decay with age: "I can remember what I had for breakfast today, but not what I had for breakfast on this day a year ago, because I have had many breakfasts since then that interfere with my ability to pick out any single one from the crowd."

HINT: #3 is astral

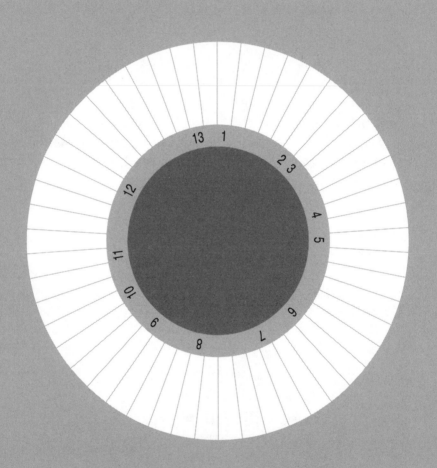

Just as one word leads to another, words lead into each other, or overlap. If you start in slot #1 with the right word, you should have little trouble completing the circle with 12 additional overlapping words. Each word starts in a numbered slot that corresponds to the number of the clue.

Clues

1. Lobe where Broca's area is
2. Unable to read, from brain damage
3. Wordbook or dictionary
4. Shaped like a Ben & Jerry receptacle
5. Addictive stimulant
6. Fortitude; impertinence; type of cell

7. Tediously loquacious
8. Old and feeble-minded
9. Kind of aid or age
10. Greek letter
11. With "over", delivered into custody
12. Part of a brain cell that receives messages
13. Diminutive mischief-maker

Starters: There are four major brain lobes: *frontal*, *temporal*, *parietal*, and *occipital*.

BRAIN BITES

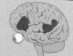

Since vocabulary size has more to do with experience and education than with raw mental agility, you might think it isn't a good measure of intelligence. But vocabulary size tends to correlate with other standard intelligence measures, such as performing math calculations or logical operations.

HINT: #12 is dendrite.

*Logic is nothing more than a knowledge
of words.*

— Charles Lamb, *Letter to Thomas Manning*, 1801

REAL-LIFE LOGIC

5 Option-Evaluation
Deductive Logic Sets
Self-Test: *Visual 20 Questions*

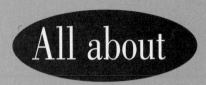
All about

REAL-LIFE
LOGIC

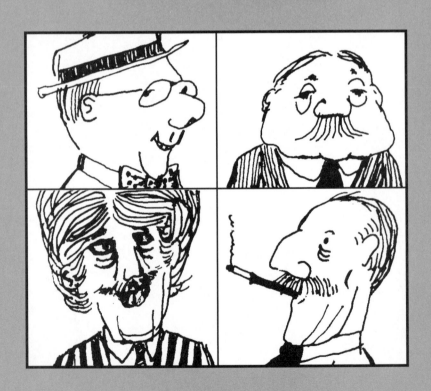

Some people think of "logic" as an academic discipline, a sub-domain of mathematics or philosophy. (There is, in fact, something called "formal logic" that you can study in college, a field with its own special symbols and language, which can get very far removed indeed from everyday life. In formal logic, for example, there is a notation for *and*, but no separate one for *but* — an important difference in real-life human attitudes but not in formal-logical expression.) On the other hand, there's a less specialized sense of the word "logic" that applies to figuring out real-life situations, such as, "If muddle-headedness can be due to a vitamin deficiency, that *doesn't* necessarily mean I'll make myself smarter by taking multivitamins." Without this kind of everyday logical acuity, we risk falling prey to snake-oil salesmen and demagogues.

The Real-Life Logic puzzles on the following pages require no specialized knowledge, technical vocabulary, or computational ability beyond basic addition, subtraction, multiplication, and division. You won't even have to remember any equations from high-school algebra. What you *will* need to do is study the facts and assumptions you're given, and use that information to come up with new information — the solution to the puzzle.

It might help to keep in mind that not all the facts in the puzzle will be equally important, or even necessary to get the answer. Sometimes, you'll begin to smell a red herring or two. But there are no trick questions. All you'll have to do is pay attention to the details of the puzzle and sort them into what's relevant and what's not. Learning to solve these logic puzzles can help in real-life situations because unwarranted assumptions lead to sloppy thinking, prejudice, and wrong conclusions.

Sometimes, you might want to draw a simple diagram to help you organize the information in the puzzle. Consider this little problem: According to your friends, Aika makes a better CD player than Electroflux, Best Brand makes a worse one than Electroflux, Cox makes a worse one than Best Brand, and Best Brand makes a better one than Daiwa; given a choice between Daiwa and Aika, which one should you choose according to your friends' opinions? (Forget about price — don't bring in criteria that aren't mentioned in the puzzle itself; remember, there are no trick questions.) The problem is confusing, but extremely simple once you order the brands left to right according to quality:

$$A > E > B > \{C, D\}$$

Now, you can see in a flash that A would be the better choice.

Another handy trick for organizing data is to draw a grid. Let's say Amy, Babette, Cleo and Dorcas are aunts of Zelda, a pragmatic woman in her 30's who decides it's about time to settle down and get married. There are four acceptable bachelors who are all eager for Zelda's hand: Ernie, Fred, Garth, and Horatio. Of course, the aunts all have opinions about which young man their niece should marry. Amy likes Ernie best and wants Zelda to marry him, Babette deems Ernie and Horatio too ugly but finds Fred and Garth worthy, Cleo likes only Garth, and Dorcas thinks Fred and Horatio are too poor but likes Ernie and Garth.

Tired of their meddling, Zelda goes to a professional matchmaker who quickly selects one of the four young men for her. Here's the puzzle: Only one of the aunts ended up being happy with the matchmaker's choice. Which aunt? And who was the lucky young man?

A confusing problem, until you lay out the aunts' choices like this (aunts on the vertical axis, men on the horizontal, with a check meaning that that aunt likes that man):

	Ernie	Fred	Garth	Horatio
Amy	✔			
Babette		✔	✔	
Cleo			✔	
Dorcas	✔		✔	

Now, you see that if only one aunt ended up being happy with the match, it must have been Babette, and the lucky young man must have been Fred. Any other choice, and either no aunt would have been happy, or more than one would have been.

Different minds work in different ways, and the best approach to a problem may depend more on the way your own mind works than on the problem itself. We have, it should be mentioned, omitted any blatantly spatial logic problems from this selection.

For those of you who are interested in pursuing formal logic or mathematics in academia, the processes of reasoning you'll use in these puzzles do come in handy in those disciplines. (More everyday logic: You don't need to know formal logic to solve these problems, but that doesn't mean that you don't need to be good at this kind of thinking to be a good formal logician.) And if you want to go to graduate school, you might like to know that the Analytical section of the GRE has questions that are similar to the puzzles here — although a lot less fun, especially at 8 a.m. in a cold gymnasium with an ill-tempered proctor pacing behind your back.

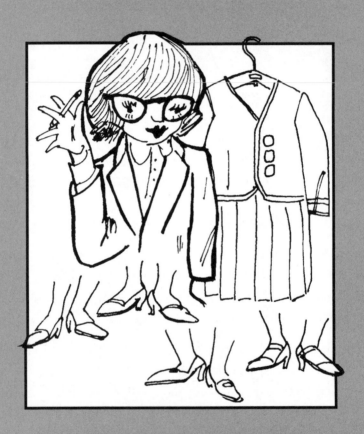

Betty was quite fashion-conscious although her working wardrobe was limited to four suits (blue with yellow, blue with aqua, blue and lavender, and blue with pink), all with matching accessories, and three pairs of shoes (all in tones of blue). She always made a nice appearance, which no doubt was one of the factors that led to her large commission checks in her new job as Outside Sales Manager. On Friday, she decided to use some of her commission money to buy a bright blue suit and shoes that matched exactly. The next Monday she wore her new outfit for the first time, then continued alternating her suits and shoes. How many days passed before the new suit and shoes were again worn together?

BRAIN BITES

If you want to win a face-to-face argument, stand toward your opponent's left side. That's the conclusion that Roger Drake at the University of Colorado drew after several carefully-designed experiments. Why? Some neuroscientists believe that the left hemisphere houses a sort of critical censor, while the right handles data in a more neutral, nonjudgmental way. So, since someone's left visual field connects to his right brain, standing to the left helps you speak more directly to his nonjudgmental right brain and bypass his left brain's critical faculty.

HINT: Since she now has 5 dresses, Betty wears her new dress every fifth weekday. But since she has only four pairs of shoes, she wears her new shoes every fourth workday. You're looking for the first workday when the new dress and the new shoes coincide.

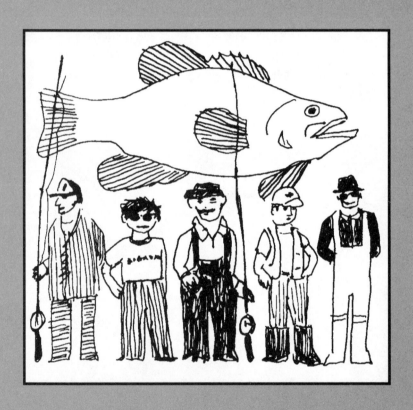

The trout season opened last week and four businessmen, Tom, Dick, Harry and Jim, along with their accountant Able, got fishing licenses. On Sunday the five men left in Dick's van for a well-stocked lake. At the end of the day Jim had caught 30 fish, twice as many as his friend Harry, whose catch amounted to 20 percent of the total taken. Able caught 10 fish. Tom and Dick took the balance between them. What was the total number of fish brought in by the five men?

BRAIN BITES

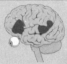

Harvard psychiatrist Fredric Schiffer has found that a simple pair of goggles, modified to block access to one brain hemisphere, has as dramatic an effect on reducing his patients' anxiety levels as pharmaceutical antidepressants, and much more quickly. (All you need is an inexpensive pair of regular plastic safety goggles and some masking tape.) EEG studies show that the goggles work by stimulating the hemisphere opposite from the unobstructed field of vision. In 60% of his patients with major depression, the goggles that block out the left visual field (connecting to the right brain) work best, indicating that their left hemisphere is their emotionally positive-minded side.

HINT: The only information you really need is in the sentence that tells you what Jim and Harry caught.

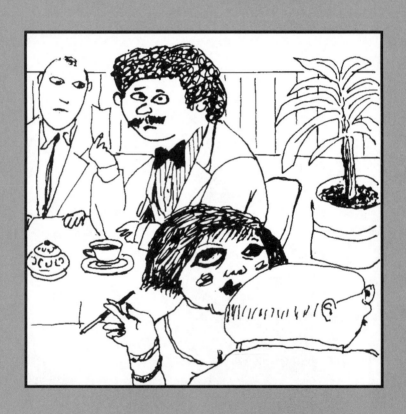

Tom and Dick recently had a late dinner at a moderately-priced restaurant after a long day spent doing the inventory at their hardware store. They were both tired and Dick paid the $45 tab without checking the arithmetic. The cashier did routine addition and discovered that the bill should have been $30. He gave the waiter three $5 bills; the waiter kept one and returned the other two to Dick. Thus Dick paid $35 for the dinners and the waiter became $5 richer, accounting for $40. What happened to the other $5?

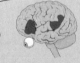

BRAIN BITES

If you're trying to follow two conversations at once, you'll do better at keeping track of the one you hear with the ear opposite from your brain's main language centers (the right ear/left hemisphere, for most people). The brain is wired so that each ear connects to both hemispheres, but, according to research by Doreen Kimura at the Montreal Neurological Institute, your brain responds to *competing* sounds by sending information from each ear to the *opposite* side of the brain.

HINT: Don't forget that the bill should have been $30, and Dick ended up paying $35.

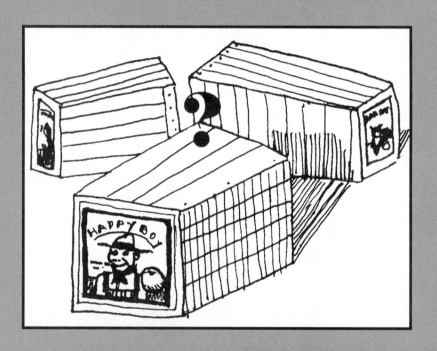

Tom and Dick recently took a vacation from their hardware store and headed south to a warmer climate. Before they left they had promised to ship a box of citrus fruit to each of their associates in the shopping complex they shared. Their cousin Harry asked for oranges, greengrocer Jim asked for pink grapefruit, and Able, the accountant, said he would like a combination of the two.

The fruit arrived a few days after Tom and Dick had returned, in boxes bearing the labels "Oranges," "Grapefruit," and "Oranges and Grapefruit." Tom then announced that he had persuaded the packer to mislabel each box, and challenged his friends to determine which box was which by taking only one piece of fruit from just one box. Able found a way to do this. Can you?

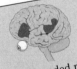

BRAIN BITES

The language-processing centers in the brains of left-handed people tend to be less exclusively located in their left hemisphere than right-handers. (Could it be that a greater integration of verbal and nonverbal areas might lead to greater creativity among lefties?) What are the chances of being born left-handed? Handedness researchers I. C. McManus and M. P. Bryden have calculated that if both parents are right-handed, about 9%. If one is right-handed, about 19%. If both are left-handed, about 26%. .

HINT: The trick is to figure out the one box whose contents can be identified by pulling out just one fruit. Remember, every box is mislabeled.

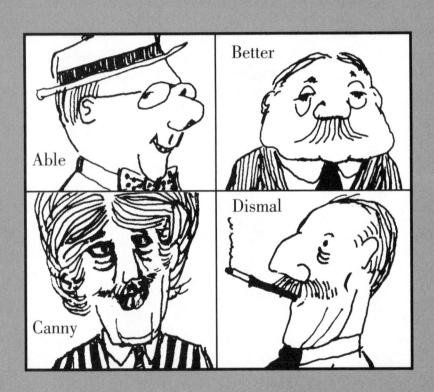

Hardware store owners Tom and Dick were considering pooling their resources with the other businesses in their shopping complex to hire a full-time accountant. Harry, the drug store owner, and Jim, who owned the greengrocery, met with Tom and Dick to interview four candidates for the position: Able (who already kept accounts for Tom and Dick), Better, Canny, and Dismal. They could not agree on the right man, so they engaged a CPA to make the decision; while they waited, they reaffirmed their choices:

Tom thought Able might be selected, but not Better or Canny.

Dick felt Better would be fine, but certainly Canny and Able were not the sort he would hire.

Harry wanted Better or Canny but not Dismal or Able.

Jim said anyone but Able would be satisfactory.

Only one made the right choice. Who was hired?

BRAIN BITES

Specific left- and right-brain differences, such as the left's specialization for language or the right's strength in visual pattern analysis, might reflect larger hemispheric differences in cognitive style. For example, neuropsychologist Elkhonon Goldberg and Louis Costa argue that the left hemisphere excels at the quick and efficient processing of data that fit familiar codes, while the right is better at dealing with novel information.

HINT: If only one made the right choice, all three of the others were wrong. Which three can be wrong without any contradiction? Work through it like this: "If Jim was wrong, then Able must have been selected," etc.

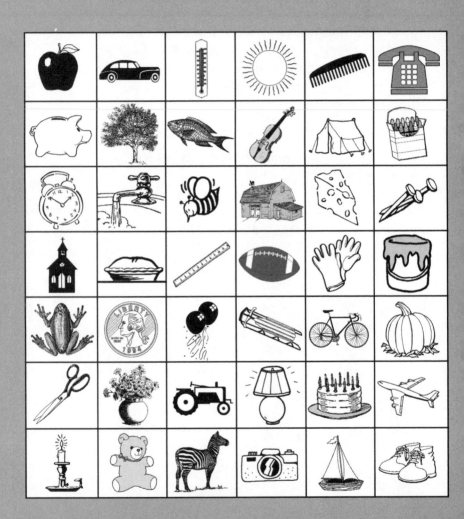

VISUAL 20 QUESTIONS

Everybody's familiar with the old parlor game of "20 Questions." One player starts out announcing whether the thing he is thinking of is "animal, vegetable, or mineral," and the other player may ask up to 20 yes-no questions to figure out the identity of the thing the first player has in mind. In this version, one player silently selects an object from the grid at the left, and the other player asks yes-no questions until he identifies the object. Then you switch roles, and the player who needs the fewest questions to get the answer wins. This game uses left-brain categorization skills (as implied by a question such as, "Is it a man-made object?"), short-term memory skills (to keep track of what you've already asked), logical thinking skills (to understand, for example, that the answer to "Is it a tool?" may eliminate the need to ask, "Is it a man-made object?"), and planning and organizational skills.

Starters: The most simple-minded strategy would be to ask, for each object in turn, "Is it the apple?" etc. For 42 squares, you'd stand only a 50-50 chance of getting the answer in 21 questions, and you might need as many as 41 questions. A better approach would be to start out with what psychologists call *constraint-seeking* questions to narrow down the possibilities, and *then* ask more specific questions to test your emerging hypothesis. A good constraint-seeking question might be, "is it bigger than my head?" or, "Is it a man-made object?" A bad one (what psychologists call *pseudo*-constraint-seeking, since it doesn't really reduce alternatives) would be, for example, "Does it have inch marks on it?"

Note, by the way, that you could take a right-brain approach to this game and apply a purely *spatial* strategy: "Is it in the right top half of the grid?" followed by, "Is it in the bottom four rows of the bottom half?" and so on until you've identified the correct square. With this method, for a 42-square grid, you'd never need more than six questions.

*The study of mathematics, like the
Nile, begins in minuteness but ends in
magnificence.* — C.C.Coulton, *Lacon*, 1820

ADDLOCKS

13 Progressively
Difficult, Deductive
Concentration Tasks

All about

ADDLOCKS

	1	2		3	4	
5				6		7
		8	9			
10		11		12		13
14	15			16	17	
	18 9	6	1	2	3	

A ddlocks are a lot like regular crossword puzzles, except that both the clues and the answers are numbers rather than words. As with crossword puzzles, the intersecting format makes it both harder and easier to come up with a correct answer. It's harder because not just any old answer of the right length will do, since intersecting answers must match. But it's also easier, since the answer to an easy clue will help you figure out a more difficult intersecting one.

For every Addlock puzzle, there are some fixed rules. Zero is never allowed. No number is ever used twice in any single answer. For example, let's say you're trying to solve 1 Across:

1	2
	3

Across
1. 6
3. 19

Down
2. 10

1 Across has two spaces, so you need two numbers that will add up to 6. In theory, there are seven possible answers: 0-6, 1-5, 2-4, 3-3, 4-2, 5-1, and 6-0. But since zero isn't allowed, you can eliminate the first and last. And since you can't have two of the same numbers in one answer, you can eliminate 3-3. That leaves you with 1-5, 2-4, 4-2, and 5-1.

Sometimes, you'll be given extra clues such as that a given number other than zero is never allowed as well. Also, we might tell you that all the answers end in an odd number, or an even number. These are important clues that will help you narrow down the field of possible answers.

Taking another look at our example, let's say we told you that 8 is never allowed in this puzzle and that all answers must end in an even number. The even-number clue rules out 1-5 and 5-1, leaving 2-4 and 4-2. Now, look at 2 Down (clue: "10"). If the answer for 2 Down began with 2, then the second number would have to be 8, which is not allowed. So you know 1 Across must be 2-4, and 2 Down must be 4-6. One answer leads to another, and you're on your way.

Since short answers are easier to solve than long ones, it's usually good to start short and work your way to long ones from there. If you look at 3 Across, a 3-number row, you'll see that the answer to 2 Down gives you the first number in 3 Across's solution. To see how easy it is to get the answer with that head start, take a moment to figure out the other possible numbers that will add up to the number given in the clue, "19." The 6 you already have tells you that you need two more numbers that must add up to 13: 9-4, 8-5, 7-6, 6-7, 5-8, or 4-9. Since 8 is not allowed and you can't have two 6's in one row, you're left with the first and last options, and since the row must end in an even number, you know only the first can be right. So of all the possible three-number series that could add up to 19, you've singled out the only possible correct answer.

¹2	²4		
	³6	9	4

Across
1. 6
3. 19

Down
2. 10

An interesting variant of the Addlock puzzle is the diagramless Addlock. This subtype is similar to a regular Addlock the way that a diagramless crossword puzzle is similar to a regular crossword. Instead of a grid with black squares filled in, you're given a blank grid and you have have to start by figuring out which squares to black out. For example, take a look at the puzzle below:

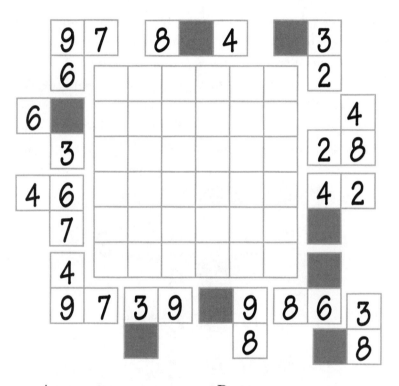

Across
1. 18 (4)   8. 20 (4)
5. 24 (3)   10. 22 (3)
6. 19 (4)   11. 21 (4)

Down
2. 21 (3)   6. 23 (4)
3. 21 (4)   10. 21 (4)
4. 22 (4)   11. 21 (3)

The first step is to use the clues to diagram the puzzle. Here's how to do it:

The number in parentheses in 1 Across tells you that answer is four digits long, so you darken the fifth square. The next clue, 5 Across, is three digits long, which won't fit on the first row. So 5 Across must go on the second row. But where? Check the "Down" clues: There's no 1 Down, so fill in a black square immediately beneath square number one. 2 Down is three digits long. But which of the squares on the first row is square number two? A hint helps: In this puzzle, no two black squares are next to each other either horizontally or vertically. So you know that the second square must be square number two, and you count down three squares from there and put a black square at the end. Continuing in this way, you complete the puzzle's pattern, and then transfer the pieces into the grid so that they fit the pattern and the clues. Here's what you end up with:

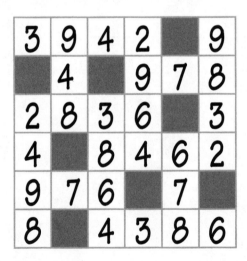

In addition to the clue that no two black squares are next to each other, it helps to remember this general rule: You should always end up with a grid diagram that is, as mathematicians say, "symmetric about its center." That means that the pattern should look the same whether you're holding the puzzle rightside-up or upside-down.

In adding this initial pattern-diagramming step to the Addlock puzzles, you might argue we're introducing a right-brain based pattern-analysis task to a left-brain puzzle book. It's interesting, though, that you can get the right answer — that is, the right pattern — by proceeding in incremental steps, using just the information contained in the clues, without really performing much pattern analysis or compositional visual processing at all. Working by the procedure described above, the patterned grid will emerge whether or not you attempt to visualize it, much as a pattern emerges in a graph you create by plotting number values onto the X and Y axes of a grid. Of course, you can always check your answer at the end by seeing if the puzzle grid has indeed ended up being symmetrical, and you can even challenge your spatial IQ by checking the grid's symmetry by rotating the pattern in your mind's eye, without moving the page.

One final note about the diagramless Addlocks: you are free, of course, to fill the numbers into the grid without looking at the pieces surrounding the grid. In fact, you'll have to work out solutions to at least some of the clues before beginning to transfer those pieces into the puzzle. Those jigsaw-like pieces therefore serve as clues or extra help in the puzzle's solution, rather than as truly necessary elements. Once you've sketched out some of the answers based on the clues, and transferred some of the pieces in, the pace of the solution will pick up as the remaining pieces fall into their places more and more rapidly.

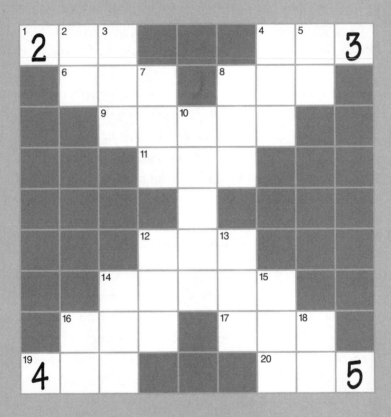

Addlocks are like crossword puzzles with interlocking numbers instead of words. Write a single digit in each box so the sum of the digits equals the total given in the clue for that row or column. No number is used more than once in any answer, and zero is not used.

In this Addlock, all answers end in an odd number.

Across

1. 7	9. 25	16. 19
4. 8	11. 22	17. 20
6. 16	12. 17	19. 20
8. 22	14. 34	20. 17

Down

2. 11	8. 20	14. 19
3. 10	10. 29	15. 24
4. 13	12. 23	16. 11
5. 13	13. 18	18. 12
7. 18		

Starters: Work from the corners in. Don't forget that no number may be repeated in an answer, and all answers must end in an odd number. Those two facts alone allow only one possible answer for 1 Across, which, in turn, leads you to one possible answer for 2 Down, and so on.

BRAIN BITES

How long would it take you to memorize a table of 50 one-digit numbers? The Russian mnemonic genius Shereshevskii need just three minutes. Quirks of his brain wiring, so to speak, gave him vivid, indelible images of all sorts of trivial data, whether he wanted them or not.

HINT: One possible answer for 6 Across is 745. 10 Down is 46829.

ADDLOCK 2

Addlocks are like crossword puzzles with interlocking numbers instead of words. Write a single digit in each box so the sum of the digits equals the total given in the clue for that row or column. No number is used more than once in any answer, and zero is not used.

In this Addlock, all answers end in an even number.

Across

1. 7   11. 16   18. 15
4. 8   12. 35   20. 20
6. 23   14. 22   21. 19
8. 24   15. 34   23. 13
9. 19   17. 18   24. 12

Down

2. 10   8. 18   16. 7
3. 21   10. 32   17. 18
4. 18   11. 29   19. 21
5. 13   13. 22   20. 13
7. 21   15. 22   22. 10

Starters: Work from the corners in. Remembering that no number may be repeated in a row, you can figure out what the numbers are in 1 Across, with only their order being uncertain. You can rule out one of those three numbers as the final one by the fact that all answers must end in an even number; 2 and 3 Down will help you eliminate other possibilities.

BRAIN BITES

Have a friend read aloud to you the first four numbers below, then repeat them back. Repeat for five numbers, and so on, until you make a mistake. What's your limit? For almost everybody, it's around six or seven.

7, 12, 3, 5, 9, 11, 5, 1, 6, 2, 8, 7, 4, 15

HINT: One possible answer for 10 Down is 49586.

Addlocks 145

ADDLOCK 3

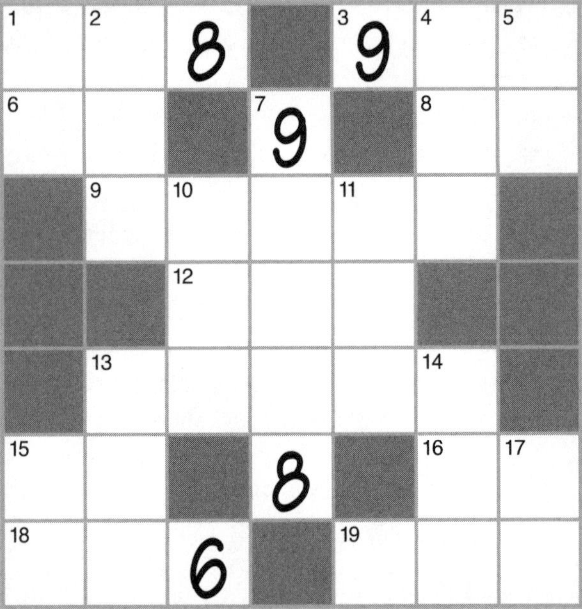

Write a single digit in each box so the sum of the digits equals the total given in the clue for that row or column. No number is used more than once in any answer, and zero is not used.
In this Addlock, all answers end in an even number; also, 3 and 4 are not used.

Across

1. 22	13. 32
3. 22	15. 15
6. 14	16. 11
8. 17	18. 16
9. 35	19. 19
12. 16	

Down

1. 11	11. 19
2. 23	13. 23
4. 24	14. 17
5. 14	15. 11
7. 31	17. 10
10. 21	

Starters: Work from the corners in. 1 Down has only one possible answer, given the restrictions stated. Therefore, 1 and 6 Across each have only one possible answer, and so does 2 Down.

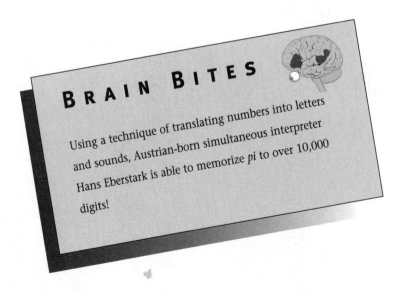

BRAIN BITES

Using a technique of translating numbers into letters and sounds, Austrian-born simultaneous interpreter Hans Eberstark is able to memorize *pi* to over 10,000 digits!

HINT: One possible answer for 7 Down is 95278.

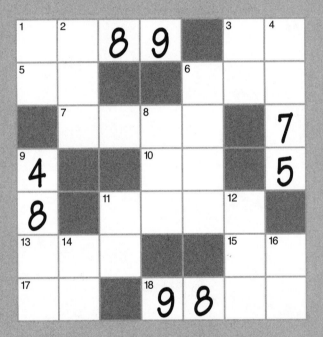

Write a single digit in each box so the sum of the digits equals the total given in the clue for that row or column. No number is used more than once in any answer, and zero is not used. In this Addlock, all answers end in an odd number.

Across

1. 30	11. 13
3. 17	13. 18
5. 8	15. 13
6. 18	17. 14
7. 23	18. 25
10. 11	

Down

1. 9	9. 28
2. 21	11. 13
3. 17	12. 12
4. 24	14. 7
8. 7	16. 12

Starters: Start with the numbers that have been partially filled in. Remembering that you can't use two of the same numbers in a row or column, you can figure out the first two numbers in 1 Across, with only their order being uncertain. Since 1 Down must end in an odd number, you can eliminate one ordering possibility for 1 Across, and you're on your way.

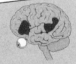

BRAIN BITES

Lack of sleep is especially harmful to mathematical ability, according to psychologist M. Mikulincer and colleagues. A study of mathematics graduates students showed that they were unable to perform even the simplest calculations if awakened from recovery sleep following a 48-hour period of sleep deprivation.

HINT: One possible answer for 6 Down is 6795.

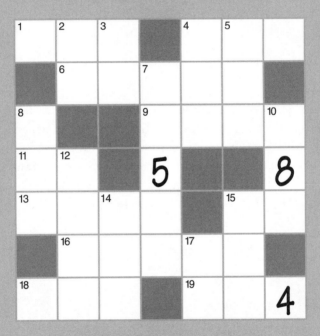

Write a single digit in each box so the sum of the digits equals the total given in the clue for that row or column. No number is used more than once in any answer, and zero is not used.
In this Addlock, all answers end in an even number, and the number 9 is not used.

Across

1.	7	13.	26
4.	8	15.	11
6.	20	16.	28
9.	25	18.	17
11.	15	19.	18

Down

2.	6	10.	18
3.	12	12.	24
4.	14	14.	19
5.	11	15.	19
7.	23	17.	15
8.	21		

Starters: The top left corner is a good place to start. Then, you can deduce the three numbers you need to complete 6 Across, with the only question being the order of the first two of those three. (Remember that all answers must end in an even digit.) 4 Down plus answers intersecting with that will help determine the order.

BRAIN BITES

Einstein was no genius at left-brain-dependent mathematical calculations. As a schoolboy, arithmetic was almost as much a struggle for him as foreign languages, and even during his residency at Princeton, after winning the Nobel Prize for physics, he had a hard time helping high-school students with their calculus homework.

HINT: One possible answer for 7 Down is 17564.

	1	6	2	3		4	5
			6		7		8
		8			9	10	
	11					12	
	13		14		15		
	8		16	17			18
	19			20		6	

Write a single digit in each box so the sum of the digits equals the total given in the clue for that row or column. No number is used more than once in any answer, and zero is not used. In this Addlock, all answers end in an odd number.

Across

1. 27	12. 14
4. 15	13. 15
6. 22	15. 13
8. 15	16. 19
9. 22	19. 12
11. 13	20. 27

Down

1. 17	10. 24
2. 19	11. 28
3. 16	14. 12
5. 29	15. 22
7. 14	17. 10
8. 20	18. 13

Starters: There's only one possible answer for 1 Down, so that's a good place to start. (Remember that all answers must end in an odd number.) From there, you can complete 1 Across, and you're on your way.

B R A I N   B I T E S

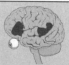

Although it's second nature to adults, young children do not automatically understand that the number-word used to count the last item in a set of items may also be used to identify the *quantity* of the set as a whole. How can you tell if your child has successfully made this conceptual jump? Just ask her to count the number of fingers on your hands. Then, ask her how many fingers you have. If she has to re-count, then she hasn't yet understood the significance of the last number-word mentioned in a counting sequence.

HINT: A good answer for 6 Across is 679.

Addlock 7

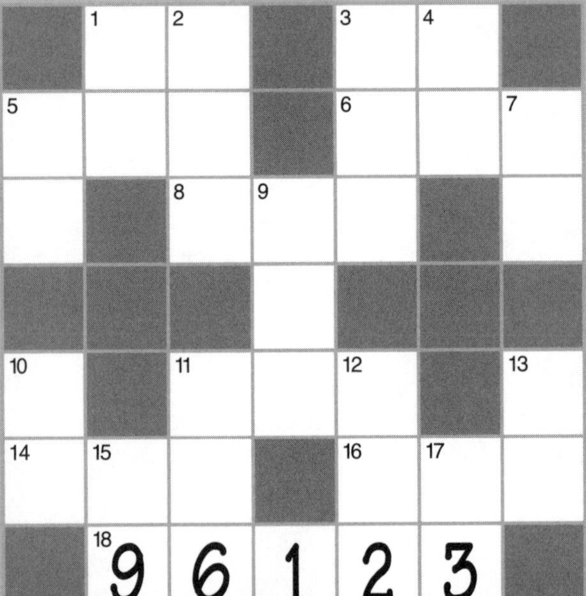

Write a single digit in each box so the sum of the digits equals the total given in the clue for that row or column. No number is used more than once in any answer, and zero is not used.

In this Addlock, every horizontal answer (but not vertical one!) ends in an odd number.

Across

1. 13	6. 16	14. 19
3. 14	8. 17	16. 20
5. 15	11. 18	18. 21

Down

1. 12	7. 9	12. 14
2. 16	9. 15	13. 8
3. 17	10. 10	15. 11
4. 13	11. 20	17. 11
5. 10		

Starters: Start at the bottom. 15 and 17 Down are good entry points. Once you solve 15 Down, 14 Across and 11 Down fall into place. 11 Across will help you single out one answer for 12 Down and, then, for 16 Across.

BRAIN BITES

Camilla Benbow has found that mathematically gifted students have a high rate of allergies. This may support Geschwind and Galaburda's theory that high testosterone levels in the womb may both harm the immune system and slow development of the left hemisphere, resulting in an accelerated growth of the right hemisphere and superior spatial skills.

HINT: This puzzle gets harder as you go up. A good answer for 2 Down is 952.

Addlocks   155

1	2	3	*8*		4	5
6				7		
	8			9		
10		11	*7*			*2*
12	13			14	15	
16				17		18
19			20			

Write a single digit in each box so the sum of the digits equals the total given in the clue for that row or column. No number is used more than once in any answer, and zero is not used.

In this Addlock, every answer ends in an even number.

Across

1. 21	9. 19	16. 14
4. 13	11. 22	17. 8
6. 21	12. 16	19. 14
7. 22	14. 15	20. 25
8. 14		

Down

1. 17	5. 20	13. 20
2. 18	7. 38	15. 9
3. 32	10. 23	18. 10
4. 24		

Starters: 1 Down is a good starting point, since there's only one possible answer (remember that every answer ends in an even digit). 11 Across is another line you can solve right away: since you're not allowed to repeat a number on a line, and every answer must end in an even number, there's only one possibility.

BRAIN BITES

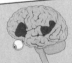

Average male superiority in spatially-based mathematics is probably partly due to biological gender differences, since cross-cultural tests show men to be somewhat superior to women in some spatial skills.

HINT: A good answer for 7 Down is 576938.

ADDLOCK 9

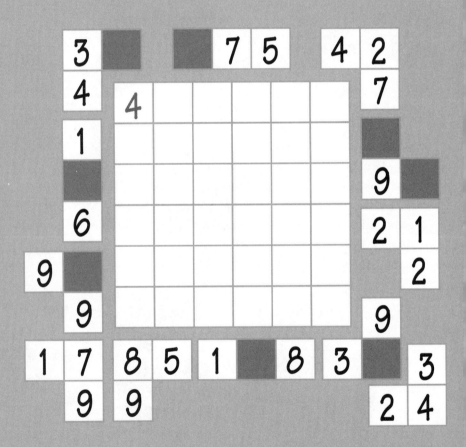

158

Solve this puzzle as you would a regular Addlock, by writing a single digit in each box so the sum of the digits equals the total given in the clue for that row or column. But first, you have to diagram the puzzle, putting in a black square at the end of each number. For instance, 1 Across is three digits, so you darken the fourth square. Looking ahead, you find that 4 Across is two digits; that takes care of the first row. In the second row, 5 Across is four digits. To help figure out exactly where to place it, check the vertical numbers and put a black square at the end of each. Clue #1 starts in upper left corner.

In this Addlock, no two black squares are adjacent. All the answers end in odd digits. As always, no number is used more than once in any answer, and zero is not used.

Across

1. 7 (3)
4. 17 (2)
5. 13 (4)
8. 13 (4)
10. 10 (4)
12. 26 (4)
14. 15 (2)
15. 21 (3)

Down

2. 9 (2)
3. 15 (5)
4. 12 (3)
6. 17 (5)
7. 10 (2)
9. 16 (2)
11. 19 (3)
13. 14 (2)

Starters: There's only one possible series of numbers for 3 Down; 1 Across helps you figure out their order. The numbers in 10 Across are certain, too. There's only one possible answer for 4 Across. We've filled in the first digit to get you started.

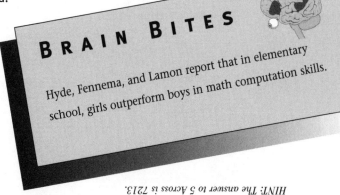

BRAIN BITES

Hyde, Fennema, and Lamon report that in elementary school, girls outperform boys in math computation skills.

HINT: The answer to 5 Across is 7213.

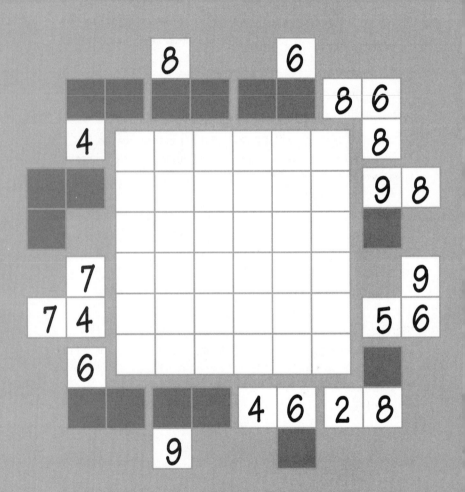

160

Solve this puzzle as you would a regular Addlock, by writing a single digit in each box so the sum of the digits equals the total given in the clue for that row or column. But first, you have to diagram the puzzle, putting in a black square at the end of each number. The clues tell you (in parentheses) how many digits are in each answer. No number is used more than once in any answer, and zero is never used.

In this Addlock, all the answers end in even digits. The design in the grid is not only symmetric about the center, but also mirror-image symmetric both vertically and horizontally.

Across

1. 17 (2)   8. 14 (2)
3. 10 (2)   9. 27 (4)
4. 30 (4)   11. 11 (2)
7. 11 (2)   12. 10 (2)

Down

2. 14 (2)   6. 25 (4)
3. 12 (2)   9. 15 (2)
5. 30 (4)   10. 6 (2)

Starters: 1 Across has only one possible answer, so that's a good place to start. That will give you the solution to 2 Down, which will lead to the solution to 4 Across.

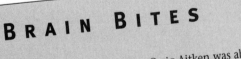

BRAIN BITES

Human calculator Alexander Craig Aitken was able to multiply any pair of three-digit numbers — say, 374 by 719 — in two seconds.

HINT: The white squares in the grid form an X. The answer to 6 Down is 7468.

ADDLOCK 11

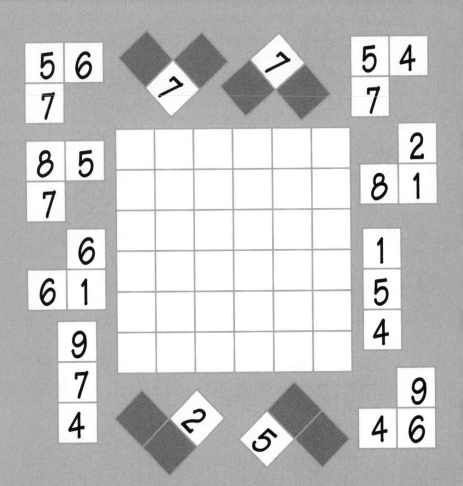

Solve this puzzle as you would a regular Addlock, by writing a single digit in each box so the sum of the digits equals the total given in the clue for that row or column. But first, you have to diagram the puzzle, putting in a black square at the end of each number. The clues tell you (in parentheses) how many digits are in each answer. No number is repeated in any answer, and zero is never used.

In this Addlock, the third and fourth lines each have two adjacent black squares.

Across

1. 16 (3)   9. 22 (4)
3. 13 (2)   12. 18 (3)
5. 13 (2)   14. 9 (2)
6. 10 (3)   15. 10 (2)
7. 21 (4)   16. 16 (3)

Down

1. 18 (3)   8. 20 (3)
2. 11 (3)   10. 20 (3)
3. 15 (2)   11. 9 (3)
4. 7 (2)   12. 9 (2)
6. 10 (3)   13. 15 (2)

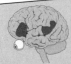

BRAIN BITES

Mathematical education researchers Benbow and Stanley tell us that in the U.S., boys start to outperform girls in math about when they reach seventh grade. Hyde and colleagues report, though, that the gender differences are shrinking.

HINT: The answer to 7 Across is 6195.

ADDLOCK 12

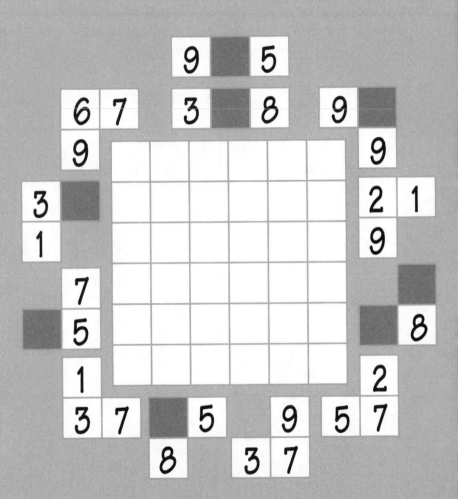

Solve this puzzle as you would a regular Addlock, by writing a single digit in each box so the sum of the digits equals the total given in the clue for that row or column. But first, you have to diagram the puzzle, putting in a black square at the end of each number. The clues tell you (in parentheses) how many digits are in each answer. No number is repeated in any answer, and zero is never used.

In this Addlock, no two black squares are adjacent either vertically or horizontally. All answers end in odd digits.

Across

1. 6 (3)
3. 17 (2)
5. 16 (2)
6. 15 (3)
7. 22 (3)
10. 22 (3)
12. 12 (3)
14. 10 (2)
16. 12 (2)
17. 18 (3)

Down

1. 11 (2)
2. 13 (3)
3. 11 (2)
4. 21 (3)
6. 21 (3)
8. 23 (3)
9. 9 (3)
11. 13 (3)
13. 9 (2)
15. 16 (2)

Starters: Start with 1 Across, continue with 1 Down and 5 Across; 3 Across also has only one possible answer.

BRAIN BITES

Neuroanatomist Sandra Witelson has performed autopsies on hundreds of cancer patients since 1977 in order to study sex differences in the *corpus callosum*, the main connecting bundle of nerve fibers that allow the two halves of the brain to communicate. She has found that, as men grow older, their corpus callosum shrinks. Women's remain the same size with age.

HINT: *The answer to 2 Down is 175.*

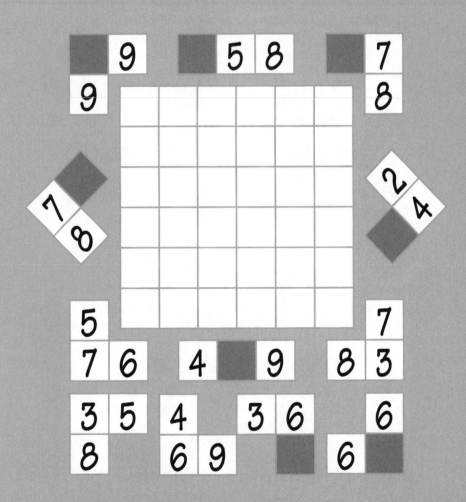

Solve this puzzle as you would a regular Addlock, by writing a single digit in each box so the sum of the digits equals the total given in the clue for that row or column. But first, you have to diagram the puzzle, putting in a black square at the end of each number. The clues tell you (in parentheses) how many digits are in each answer. No number is repeated in any answer, and zero is never used.

In this Addlock, no two black squares are adjacent either vertically or horizontally. All answers end in even digits.

Across

1. 12 (3)	9. 33 (5)
3. 11 (2)	10. 10 (2)
5. 13 (2)	12. 14 (2)
7. 30 (5)	13. 23 (3)

Down

1. 11 (2)	7. 17 (2)
2. 25 (5)	8. 9 (2)
4. 12 (3)	9. 24 (3)
6. 30 (5)	11. 15 (2)

Starters: 9 Down and 7 Down each have only one possible answer, so they're a good place to start.

BRAIN BITES

Left-handers are disproportionately gifted in mathematics, according to researchers Benbow, Witelson, Geschwind, and Galaburda. The two hemispheres in the brains of left-handers tend to be less lateralized (left-or-right-specialized). They may enjoy an advantage because the clusters of cells that process mathematical computations in their brains are distributed more widely over both hemispheres.

HINT: The answer to 2 Down is 45736.

Imagination and memory are but one thing, which for divers considerations hath divers names.

— Thomas Hobbes, *Leviathan*, VOL II, 1651

The one who thinks over his experiences most, and weaves them into systematic relations with each other will be the one with the best memory.

— William James, *Psychology, Briefer Course*, CH XVIII, 1892

LEFT-HEMI MEMORY

5 Exercises in Visual Probability
Self-Test: *Hypnotizability Scale*

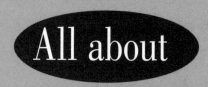

All about

LEFT-HEMI
MEMORY

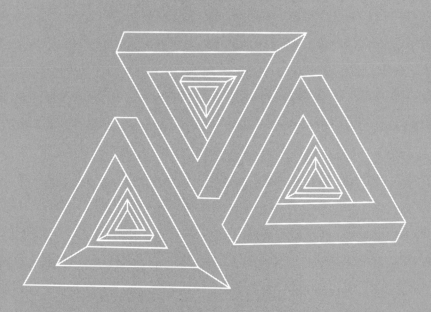

Both sides of your brain work together to remember things — sometimes inaccurately. If you want to draw something accurately, according to author Betty Edwards' "right-brain" approach, you first have to lose your left-brain preconceptions about the way what you're drawing *should* look like and reproduce only what is in front of your eyes. The left brain houses what neuroscientist Michael Gazzaniga has called an "interpreter" mechanism, while the right brain sees things more like they really are. So if you're viewing data with the right side of your brain, you're using the more *neutral* side, despite what people say about the right brain being more creative.

But what if you want to *remember* something? Gazzaniga points out that "our brains are built to remember the gist of things, not the details." So if you want to remember something, *make it meaningful* by noting how it relates to something else you know. It's the left brain, by his research, that focuses on subjective meaning, while the right brain is more literal and detail-oriented.

Sometimes the left brain may work so hard to make something meaningful out of neutral data that it alters the facts. For example, read through this list of words, then cover up the list and write down as many of the words as you can remember:

bed, slumber, dream, drowsy, pillow,
tired, nap, yawn, doze, snore

Chances are, you'll remember not only some of the words on the list, but also one word that isn't there: *sleep.* The fact that the words form a thematic group makes them easier to remember than just a random assortment of words, but it also makes it more likely that you'll falsely substitute a word fitting the theme that isn't really there.

That little self-test illustrates a simple but important fact: memory is not an objective tape-recording of the data of life, but a highly subjective *creative* process that draws as much on preconceptions and general knowledge about how the world *should* work as on the facts "out there" *in* the world. As pioneering memory researcher F. C. Bartlett phrased it in 1932: "Memory of an event reflects a blend of information retrieved from a specific trace of that event with knowledge, expectations, and beliefs derived from other sources."

Recent findings from brain-damaged and split-brain patients, and from PET scan studies of normal healthy adults, indicate that those "other sources" often reside in the left brain. Gazzaniga and Yale researcher Elizabeth Phelps have shown that it's the left hemisphere that often adds seemingly "logical" embellishments to memories. Gazzaniga and fellow Dartmouth cognitive scientist Michael Miller used PET scans to reveal that the left side of the brain becomes more active during recollections of false memories. And memory researcher Daniel Schacter has reported on a patient with right frontal lobe damage who is particularly free in creating false memories, since that part of his right brain isn't available for "reality checks."

Elizabeth Loftus, a psychologist at the University of Washington, is probably the best-known researcher on the malleability, and fallibility, of human memory. Her expert testimony has been used in several court cases in which a parent, teacher, or caretaker has been accused of molesting a child. The problem is, the preponderance of evidence indicates that young children are highly suggestible and responsive to the perceived desires of the interrogator. As Schacter has pointed out, young children are not as able as adults to sort out just what the source is of some thought or image that has entered their heads and become mixed with other memories. It's not their fault. Frontal lobe regions of the brain responsible for "source memory" — that is, remembering where and when and how a memory or image entered one's mind — are relatively undeveloped in young children. So original memories are mixed with other more recently-introduced images, becoming changed or overwritten in the process, and the children often simply don't know they're not telling the truth. (This isn't necessarily to say that children under such circumstances are not telling the truth; it's just that there are a lot of "false positives.")

We all suffer from these mix-ups to some degree, even once our frontal lobes have developed to an adult level. Loftus once designed a simple but ingenious experiment to test the theory that the brain preserves unaltered memories in some dark recess of itself. If someone sees a person reading a yellow book, and is later asked, "Did you see the person reading the blue book?", the original memory is likely to be revised. When re-questioned well after the fact, the witness will tend to supply the incorrect information that the person was reading a blue book. But if an original, accurate memory continued to coexist with the altered one, Loftus reasoned, this knowledge should come out if the witness is pressed to guess what *other* color the book "might have been." In fact, three times as many subjects in this experiment guessed the color next to blue on the spectrum — green — than guessed yellow.

lake

river

bank

ocean

shore

rocks

lighthouse

telescope

calendar

sundial

clock

watch

time

Take about a minute to study the list of words to the left. Then, cover up the list, do something else for a few minutes, and try to answer these questions:

1) Can you remember a word beginning with *w*?
   (Hint: "look.")
2) Can you remember a word beginning with *b*?
   (Hint: "savings.")

If you couldn't remember one or both of the words, try to answer the two questions below:

1) Can you remember a word from the list beginning with *w*?
   (Hint: "timepiece.")
2) Can you remember a word from the list beginning with *b*?
   (Hint: "water's edge.")

Which was easier? In the second version of the questions, the hints help you to recreate the same context of meaning that was active when you studied the words on the list, thus activating the left-brain semantic memory system in the appropriate way.

BRAIN BITES

Memory researchers Endel Tulving and Donald Thomson formulated this *encoding specificity principle* that explains one important factor bearing on our ability to remember things: "The probability of remembering an event is a function of the extent to which cues processed at the time of encoding are also processed at the time of retrieval."

Thomas wore a funny mustache.

Harold painted a starry night.

Sandra liked to wear berets.

Tim didn't want to give up the tapes.

Leonard was a brilliant theoretical physicist.

Melvin had an inspiring dream about
racial equality.

Martin had an inspiring dream about
racial equality.

Albert was a brilliant theoretical physicist.

Richard didn't want to give up the tapes.

Monica liked to wear berets.

Vincent painted a starry night.

Adolf wore a funny mustache.

First, read through the rightside-up statements on the top half of the opposite page. Then, cover them up and try to answer the following questions:

Who wore a funny mustache?
Who painted a starry night?
Who liked to wear berets?
Who didn't want to give up the tapes?
Who was a brilliant theoretical physicist?
Who had an inspiring dream about racial equality?

Check your answers and make a note of how many you got right. Next, turn the book upside-down and read through the statements on the bottom half of the opposite page. Try to answer the questions again. How many did you get right this time?

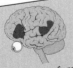

BRAIN BITES

Memory is not a camera. Facts that cohere with or are reinforced by pre-existing knowledge about the world are easier to remember than random ones. Another way your memory isn't like a camera: You'll remember a face better if you make a subjective judgment about the likability of the person behind it. So showed psychologists Bower and Karlin in a study published in 1974.

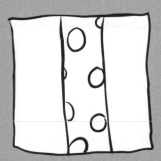

Giraffe outside
my window.

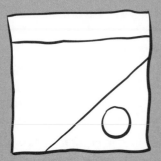

Picnic on
the moon.

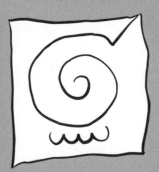

Kitten on
the keys.

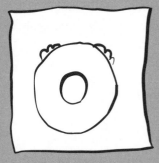

Siesta down on
the sidewalk.

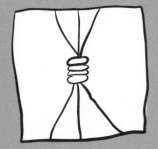

Pocket pool.

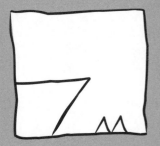

Ship arriving too late to
save a drowning cat.

Study the doodles at the left for about a half-minute each, paying attention to the titles beneath them. Then, cover them up with a blank piece of paper and try to reproduce them as faithfully as possible, prompted by the titles listed below.

Ship Arriving Too Late to Save a Drowning Cat
Giraffe Outside My Window
Siesta Down on the Sidewalk
Picnic on the Moon
Pocket Pool
Kitten on the Keys

BRAIN BITES

Memory researcher Elizabeth Loftus has demonstrated how the wording of a question can influence the answer you'll get. In an experiment of hers, people who were asked, "Do you get headaches frequently, and if so, how often?" gave an average answer of 2.2 a week. If the wording was, "Do you get headaches occasionally, and if so, how often?" the average answer was only 0.7 a week. Her research has brought about changes in guidelines police interrogators must adhere to when questioning witnesses in criminal cases.

MEMORY 4

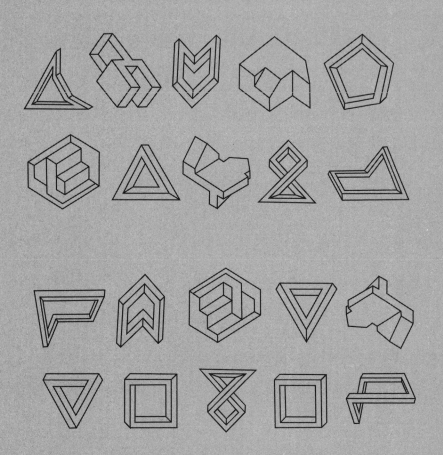

On the opposite page, cover up the lower group of ten shapes and study the upper group. For each shape, judge as rapidly as you can whether the shape is "possible" or not — whether it represents a shape that could exist in real 3-dimensional space.

After you've done that, turn the book upside-down and make the same judgments about the shapes in the lower group, again working as rapidly as possible.

Once you've done this, note that two of each of the "possible" and "impossible" shapes were repeated from the first group. Did you come to a faster conclusion about those shapes the second time around? Experiments by Daniel Schacter and Lynn Cooper have shown that people come to a judgment about the "possible" shapes more quickly if they'd already seen them the first time around — but not about the "impossible" ones. This shows that we retain memories of unfamiliar objects once we encounter them, but only if they have a consistent overall structure.

BRAIN BITES

You might think that a visual memory task like this would primarily involve the right hemisphere, but that's not quite true. In a PET scan study, Schacter and colleagues showed that when the brain is judging a new shape, there's activation in the area where the right temporal and occipital lobes meet, mostly on the right side. When re-encountering a "possible" shape (but not an "impossible" one), the left side lights up as well. In a *perceptual priming* task like this one, then, the retained visual image primes a quick judgment of a shape on a second encounter. This effect even works with amnesics.

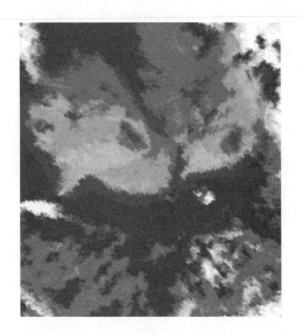

To the left is an upside-down picture of an object. Before you turn the book upside-down to see if you can tell what the object is, read the word here: *fluffy*. Now, turn the book upside-down, and after you've done that read the rest of the instructions below.

If you still had a hard time figuring out what's in the picture, take a look at the *HINT* in the small box at the bottom of the page, and then look at the picture again. Now, do you recognize what it is?

BRAIN BITES

When you try to recognize a hard-to-see visual object, it helps if your recognition is "primed" by a clue in the *same modality* as the object. For a visual object, a simple line drawing usually works better than a word. Memory works in a similar way. Endel Tulving's *encoding specificity principle* states that the likelihood of recalling an event is increased if a retrieval cue matches the way you were thinking about the event as it happened. Something like this is happening when you have a hard time matching a name to a face that you're seeing outside of its usual context (when you unexpectedly encounter a co-worker in a restaurant on the weekend, for example).

:LNIH

CREATIVE IMAGINATION
HYPNOTIZABILITY AND SUGGESTIBILITY

Dartmouth brain researcher Michael Gazzaniga points out that your left brain sometimes overinterprets events to create false memories. For example, it's quite common to get a good idea from something you read and then to remember it as an idea you came up with yourself — especially if you can convince yourself that the good new idea is consistent with what you already thought. This kind of unintentional plagiarism happens automatically and unconsciously.

The left brain's "interpreter" very likely interacts with other brain mechanisms that also help blur the distinction between fact and fantasy — for example, your power of visual imagination, in which your right hemisphere plays an important role. Memory researchers Loftus, Levidow, and Duensing have found that artists and architects are especially liable to integrate misleading suggestions into their memories. So are young children. People who are most likely to create false memories in response to misinformation tend to score higher in tests that rate their ability to produce vivid visual imagery on demand, such as the Creative Imagination Scale (Wilson and Barber 1978), a scale which can also be used to estimate your hypnotizability. Some researchers have also found that measures of your need for social approval (for example, the Social Desirability Scale of Crown and Marlowe) can help predict how hypnotizable, and suggestible, you'll be. Psychobiologist Robert Cloninger at Washington University in St. Louis views *reward dependence* (his name for the equivalent of the "social desirability" parameter in his system) as varying with your brain levels of the neurotransmitter *norepinephrine*, which interacts largely with the right hemisphere.

For this self-test (an adaptation of part of Wilson and Barber's Creative Imagination Scale), you will need a helper to play the role of "hypnotist" by slowly reading the following segments of text aloud as you concentrate with your eyes closed on what you hear.

PART ONE: "For this first part, please close your eyes and sit in a relaxed position. Place your left hand in your lap with the palm facing up.

Imagine that Novocain is being injected into the little finger of your left hand. You feel the slight prick of the needle in the tip of your little finger and then your finger starts to tingle like when you sleep on your arm or when some part of your body falls asleep. You feel your little finger tingle, and then you feel the very tip start to go numb. Imagine the Novocain moving up your finger, as first the tip goes numb, and then the first knuckle, and then the second knuckle, and then your whole little finger is numb all the way to where it meets your hand. Now, the whole little finger on your left hand is completely numb, like a fat lump of clay.

Now imagine the Novocain moving into your next finger, the ring finger, as it starts to feel numb as well. Tell yourself that this next finger is feeling number and number, until it too feels like a lump of clay, or a fat piece of rubber. Now, both fingers are numb, fat, and rubbery.

Now, bend your thumb over and feel the two fingers at the other end of your hand. Those fingers are so numb that they can't really feel the thumb touching them, just a dull sensation of pressure.

Now, tell yourself you've just imagined the whole thing, and your fingers feel perfectly normal, and not numb at all, and you can feel sensations in them perfectly fine."

PART TWO: "For this second part, lie down on your back someplace comfortable, with your head turned to the left so your right cheek is up. Close your eyes again as you listen to the instructions.

Picture yourself lying on a sun-scorched desert-island beach somewhere near the equator in the middle of the Indian Ocean. You can feel the gritty sand against your left cheek as you lie on your back with your right check turned upwards towards the scorching tropical sun. Picture the sun's hot rays caressing your right cheek and let yourself feel the heat.

As you imagine the tropical sun shining with blinding brightness, let yourself feel

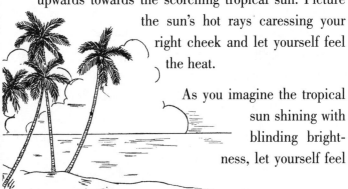

the heat increasing. Feel the sun getting hotter and hotter, burning through your skin to the cheekbone and teeth beneath. Feel the heat going deeper and deeper, so hot it's almost like radioactivity.

Feel your right cheek getting hotter. Imagine the sunburn you'll have, as the scorching noonday sun turns your right cheek redder and redder, hotter and hotter. Tell yourself the sun is penetrating into the really deep layers of skin on your right cheek, where it will make blisters bubble up, but don't turn your head, keep it turned so the right cheek is turned up to the tropical sun.

Feel your right cheek get hotter and hotter. Feel the rays of the sun going deeper. Feel your cheek get so hot that if a drop of water fell on it, it would sizzle.

Now, picture a wave coming up from the sea and washing over you, cooling you down. Tell yourself that you imagined the whole thing, and that your cheek is perfectly cool. Just remain lying there, and keep your eyes closed."

PART THREE: "For this third part, remain lying down. Keep your eyes closed as you listen to the instructions.

Imagine yourself lying by a lake in Northern Italy. There's a carpet of warm, fragrant grass beneath you. It's a beautiful summer day, with a warm sun shining out of a robin's-egg-blue sky. A gentle breeze caresses your face. Picture the blue sky with a few small, cottony clouds floating slowly by, and feel the warm sun on your face and neck. In the distance you hear a small child laugh.

Feel the gentle warmth of the sun soothe your shoulders

and chest as you lie on the soft grass. The breeze caresses the backs of your hands, and then you notice how warm and pleasant the sun feels on them. Your shoulders, arms, and hands feel so relaxed in the warm sun and gentle breeze. Small, brightly-colored sailboats drift lazily on the blue lake.

Tell yourself that you've never felt so relaxed, as the warmth of the sun flows down your arm and through your fingers, down your chest to your stomach and legs. Just let yourself go limp. The smell of the warm grass is so relaxing, so soothing. Let yourself feel the warmth of the sun as every muscle in your body melts into complete relaxation. Even your toes feel warm, calm, at peace with the grass, the water lapping at the lake's shore, the blue sky, the universe. Just let yourself feel calm, relaxed, so lazy you might never get up.

Now, open your eyes and let yourself continue to feel relaxed, but awake and alert at the same time. You may get up if you wish."

SCORING:

1. In the first part, you were asked to imagine that first your little finger and then the second finger on your left hand were turning numb from a shot of Novocain. Compared to what you would have felt if your finger really had been injected with Novocain, what you felt was:

> Not at all the same (0 pt.)
>
> A little the same (1 pt.)
>
> Somewhat the same (2 pts.)

Much the same (3 pts.)
Exactly the same (4 pts.)

2. In the second part, you were asked to imagine that you were lying on the beach on a tropical island, with the sun burning your right cheek. Compared to what you would have felt if you really had been lying on a tropical beach with the hot sun burning your cheek, what you felt was:

Not at all the same (0 pt.)
A little the same (1 pt.)
Somewhat the same (2 pts.)
Much the same (3 pts.)
Exactly the same (4 pts.)

3. In the third part, you were asked to imagine that you were lying by a peaceful Italian lake, with a warm sun and gentle breeze making you feel completely relaxed. Compared to what you would have felt if you really had ben relaxing by an Italian lake, what you felt was:

Not at all the same (0 pt.)
A little the same (1 pt.)
Somewhat the same (2 pts.)
Much the same (3 pts.)
Exactly the same (4 pts.)

Totals: 0-3 pts.: Low hypnotizability
4-7 pts.: Average hypnotizability
8-12 pts.: High hypnotizability

Everything is possible, including the impossible and absurd.

— Benito Mussolini, A Speech in Trieste, September 20, 1920

7	2	3	8	4
3	4	9	2	6
8	3	5	7	1
4	8	1	6	5
2	7	6		

DIGI-CLUES

7 Mathematical
Pattern Finders

All about

DIGI-CLUES

Number-pattern problems similar to our Digi-Clues are a standard part of many intelligence test batteries (e.g., the Stanford-Binet Number Series section). Number series with implicit patterns are also one of the things included in attempts (in real science and science fiction) to communicate with extraterrestrial life. It's assumed that any truly intelligent being, human or not, will be able to decipher them.

The most straightforward puzzles of this type present you with a series of numbers that have a single regular relationship between them. For example:

$$1 \quad 2 \quad 4 \quad 8 \ldots$$

or

$$1 \quad 5 \quad 9 \quad 13 \ldots$$

You can continue the first series simply by doubling each number as you go along; the second, by adding 4 to each number. What makes these easy is that each number in the series is the result of a single simple mathematical operation performed on the previous one, resulting in a transparently regular pattern.

Now, take a look at this:

$$7 \, 2 \, 8 \, 6 \, 4$$
$$3 \, 3 \, 5 \, 2 \, 8$$
$$5 \, 9 \, 1 \, 5 \, 8$$
$$1 \, 8 \, 7 \, 1 \, \underline{?}$$

Even with three rows of numbers to help you deduce the pattern, this is harder because there's no simple, transparent relationship between the individual numbers. Once you group some of the numbers into two-digit pairs, the problem becomes absurdly easy; the pattern can be illustrated as follows:

$$72 - 8 = 64$$

So the missing number on the fourth line is 1. The leap of insight leading you to combine numbers into two-digit pairs requires a little more than just finding a regular pattern between individual one-digit numbers.

The more kinds of operations involved (addition, division, etc.), the more challenging the puzzle will be to solve. Take a look at this one:

$$37 \quad 15 \quad 26$$
$$83 \quad 71 \quad 77$$
$$12 \quad 186 \quad 99$$
$$52 \quad 18 \quad \underline{?}$$

The job of combining single numbers into multiple-digit numbers is already done for you. But again, if you're looking for a single constant relationship between adjacent numbers in the series, you'll fail to find it.

The solution? For each line, just add the first two numbers together, and the third number is half that total. The missing number on the fourth line, then, is 35. Once you see the pattern the puzzle seems ludicrously simple. The fact, however, that you have to do two things to the first two numbers — add and then divide by two — to get the third obscures the pattern and makes the puzzle harder.

Also tricky are puzzles where a number that isn't even shown in the series provides the key to the solution. Here's an example:

$$16 \ 18 \ 19$$
$$22 \ 70 \ 77$$
$$7 \ 9 \ 1$$
$$100 \ 50 \ \underline{?}$$

What's the pattern? If you add the first two numbers together, and subtract the third from that sum, you'll always get 15. Once someone tells you, you'll slap your hand to your forehead, but there are two things that make the pattern hard to find. First, there are two operations involved. Second, you have to come up with a fourth number, in addition to the operations, to make sense of the series. But patterns that are hard to find are also more rewarding once you find them.

One final tip: sometimes, the pattern may lie vertically, not (or not just) horizontally.

1	1	2	3
5	8	13	21

Study the pattern in the squares to the left, then fill in the bottom line by writing the correct number in each box.

Starters: Have you noticed that the numbers grow larger as they progress from left to right and from the last number in one line to the first number in the next? In fact, the number in the lower right corner box has three digits.

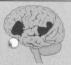

BRAIN BITES

German scientist Werner Wittling showed a romantic movie scene to either the right or left visual field of experimental subjects. In the left visual field, connecting directly to the right brain, the subjects had a significant increase in blood pressure. Other films with both positive and negative content also triggered a stronger emotional response when shown to the right hemisphere. So is the right hemisphere the "emotional" side? Some scientists think so, but others disagree. Researchers Gainotti, Caltagirone, and Zoccolotti find that the right hemisphere seems to connect more directly to brain structures (such as the primitive amygdala) that generate a basic emotional reaction while the left hemisphere plays a role of regulating or controlling the reaction. They speculate that language development in the left brain may give rise to this mediating role, rather than the left brain simply being emotionally less well-endowed.

HINT: The first number on the final line is 34.

7	2	3	8	4
3	4	9	2	6
8	3	5	7	1
4	8	1	6	5
2	7	6		

While the numbers in the grid to the left might appear to be randomly placed, there's a definite logic to their locations. Can you find the key and fill in the two missing numbers in the last row?

Starters: Work horizontally *and* vertically. If you have a sharp eye for digits, you will notice that no number appears more than once in the same row or column.

BRAIN BITES

Some people have claimed that "intuition" resides in the right hemisphere, and that women are more intuitive and right-hemisphere-dominant. In fact, it may be that the "intuitive" abilities of women come from better conscious (and verbal) *access* to their right brain's thoughts and feelings. Neuroscientists Sandra Witelson and Laura Allen and neuroendocrinologist Roger Gorski have noted gender differences in the *corpus callosum*, the main bundle of nerve fibers connecting the brain's right and left halves. Also, women tend to be less *lateralized* in their brain centers (including language centers), so information may not have to traverse their brain's divide as much as in men.

HINT: The number in the bottom right-hand corner is 8.

3	1	6	2	5
4	2	7	3	5
5	3	9	4	4
6	9	7	6	2
7	8	5		3

Can you find the pattern in this seemingly random arrangement
of numbers and fill in the empty square in the bottom row?

Starters: Work horizontally. In each row, there are two two-
digit numbers.

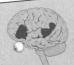

BRAIN BITES

When R. C. Oldfield distributed a handedness inventory to over
1,000 students at the University of Edinburgh in Scotland, it turned
out that the smaller left-handed group was not a simple mirror
image of the right-handed group. Most right-handers show a much
more consistent across-the-board preference for using their right
hand for most activities like writing, throwing, and brushing teeth. A
smaller number tend to show a mixed and somewhat weaker preference for using their left hand, with very few left-handers clustering
towards the extreme of consistent left-hand preference. (Right-handers also tend to be more strongly left-hemisphere dominant for language.) It's because of findings like these that some researchers
describe handedness in the population in terms of "right-handers"
and "non-right-handers," rather than "left-handers."

*HINT: Group the numbers in the first and second column
into a two-digit number, and do the same for columns
four and five; then, compare these two numbers.*

A	B	C
108	356	124
196	780	292
284	648	

On the left are two rows of three numbers each. Can you figure out the logical sequence of these numbers and fill in the final box in the third row?

Starters: Work horizontally. Do something to A and B to make C.

B R A I N   B I T E S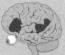

If you were asked to memorize a list of letters, and then asked to look at a picture of an object and decide whether the first letter of the object's name was among the letters memorized, you'd be using left-brain regions to make that decision. However, if you had to do it the other way around — memorize pictures of several objects, and then look at a letter and decide whether any of the memorized objects start with that letter — you'd be primarily activating your right hemisphere. This isn't just theoretical speculation. In carefully-designed experiments by Klatzky and Atkinson, subjects respond more quickly in a task such as the first one when the stimulus (the object) is flashed in the subject's right visual field, which links directly to the left hemisphere, and only indirectly to the right through the *corpus callosum* (the nerve fibers that carry signals from one hemisphere to the other). This pattern is reversed in a task such as the second one, with the flashed stimulus being a letter. So it's not so much the stimuli themselves — pictures and letters — that determine which hemisphere is more engaged, but what you *do* with them.

HINT: Start by comparing the difference between A and B to the number in column C.

6	4	8	6	4
9	3	52	24	64
16	5	66	7	

Can you find the logical sequence in these numbers and fill in the final box?

Starters: Work horizontally. Do something to the first two boxes, then the same thing to the next two. Relate them to get the answer in the fifth box.

BRAIN BITES

Harvard neuroscientist Alvaro Pascual-Leone has discovered a new treatment for depression. He places a pulsating electromagnet over the left side of the patient's head, which increases the activity of the left brain. In 60% of his patients, the treatment reduces the symptoms of depression. Since the electromagnet's pulse rate can be raised or lowered to stimulate or suppress brain activity, more studies are being done using different pulse rates on different areas of the brain.

HINT: Addition and subtraction figure prominently in this puzzle.

3	9	2	5	4
4	3	8	9	6
7	2	7	9	8
5	5	3	7	5
6	3	4		2

Study these numbers until you find the pattern and can fill in the blank square.

Starters: Work horizontally.

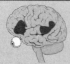

BRAIN BITES

Memory researcher Larry Squire has cited PET scan evidence that the largely unconscious aspect of memory referred to as *priming* relies mostly on the right hemisphere. (An example of priming might be completing a partially filled-in word to match a word you were shown earlier — even though you have no recollection of having seen it the first time around.) Conscious recollection of the sort sometimes referred to as *declarative* memory (such as remembering where and when you encountered the word previously) are handled by wider areas of the brain, including in the left half.

HINT: Addition is not required.

8	4	7
3	9	2
7	5	10
	6	5

Each of the top three horizontal rows of numbers follows the same mathematical pattern. Can you figure out the system and fill in the missing number in the bottom row?

Starters: What makes this Digi-Clues puzzle harder than the others is that you need to do something to the numbers in each row to get a fourth number that doesn't appear in any of the rows; that fourth number is constant from row to row.

BRAIN BITES

All human cultures add and subtract, but number systems and "tagging" conventions vary. ("Tagging" refers to routines for keeping track of counting by, say, extending the fingers in a certain order.) The Oksapmin tribe of New Guinea begin with the thumb of the right hand and end with the thumb on the left, but only after traversing 19 points up the right arm, across the shoulders and head, and then down the left arm.

HINT: Start by multiplying the first two numbers together.

He who has heard the same thing told by 12,000 eye-witnesses has only 12,000 probabilities, which are equal to one strong probability, which is far from certainty.

— Voltaire, *Philosophical Dictionary*, 1764

A reasonable probability is the only certainty.

— E. W. Howe, *Sinner Sermons*, 1926

PROBLEMATICS

5 Counter-Intuitive
Probability Deductions

All about

PROBLEMATICS

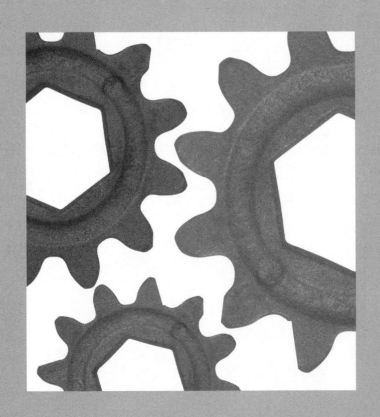

There are some kinds of left-brain logic problems that almost everybody has a hard time with. Often they seem paradoxical, counterintuitive, or just plain unapproachable from a common-sense perspective. And that's just the point. You have to suspend everyday assumptions in order to get the right answer. So if you can't do these puzzles, you don't have to feel stupid. But if you *can* solve them, you deserve to feel good about yourself, since you're succeeding at something that's hard for everybody.

For example, there's a logic problem (devised by Peter Wason) that has been used to illustrate how poor most of us are in our reasoning abilities. Imagine I lay 4 cards in front of you. The first card has "A" on it, the second "B", the third "2", the fourth "3". Each card has a number on one side and a letter on the other. You have to figure out which two cards to turn over in order to determine whether the following rule is true or false for this set of 4 cards: If a card has an "A" on one side, it has a "2" on the other. Try it, then read on.

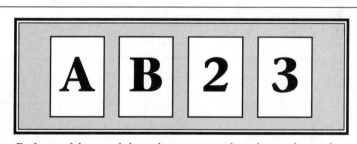

Each one of these cards has a letter on one side and a number on the other. Which two cards would you turn over in order to determine whether the following rule is true or false: If a card has an A on one side, it has a 2 on the other.

Almost everybody turns over the first card, the one with an "A" on one side. Most people also turn over the third card — card "2" — but very few people turn over card "B" or "3". Is this the right strategy? As far as the first card goes, yes: if anything other than a "2" is on the other side of the "A" then the rule is disconfirmed. But what will the third card tell you? It has "2" on one side. If you flipped it over and it had an "A" on the other side, it would provide no counterevidence to the claim. If it had something other than an "A" — say, a "Z" — then it would also provide no counterevidence. Remember, the rule is that if a card has "A" on one side, then it has "2" on the other, not that if it has "2" on one side it has an "A" on the other. So the third card is, so to speak, harmless — it cannot serve to disprove the rule, or, therefore, to test its validity. On the other hand, what about the fourth card, the one with a "3"? If you turned it over and it had an "A" on the other side, it would immediately disprove the rule. So that's the one to turn over, in addition to the first card. But very few people choose this strategy.

Once you translate the problem into less abstract terms, it's much easier to solve. Imagine you're a state trooper responsible for enforcing smog emission requirements: Everyone with a car built after 1972 must have a valid smog certification sticker.

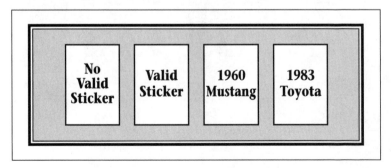

| No Valid Sticker | Valid Sticker | 1960 Mustang | 1983 Toyota |

Substitute this kind of data onto the cards, which now have information on one side about whether a car has a valid sticker or not, and information on the other about how old the car is. Which cards would you turn over to make sure the law is being complied with?

This time, you'd have no trouble correctly picking the first and last cards. There's some evidence that the right brain has some capacity to solve the problem when it's phrased this way. Of course, it would be nice to know how to solve both versions, since that gives you more flexibility. College entrance exams don't offer you the option of choosing your own format.

Even in real-life situations, we humans often have problems with logic, especially with ones involving judgments of probability. Say Mark McGuire gets an average of a hit every third at-bat — a little under two hits a game. It's the bottom of the ninth, with the game tied and a runner on second. He's had four at-bats so far in the game, and hasn't yet gotten a hit. The play-by-play announcers are talking about how "he's due." Your friend has a hunch McGuire's going to get a hit, and wants to put some money on it. Should you take the bet?

Based purely on the statistical probabilities, you'd be wise to put money against it. Since McGuire gets a base hit about one in three at-bats, he has only a one-in-three chance of getting a hit any given time at the plate. The fact that he hasn't gotten a hit yet in the game has no bearing on whether he'll get a hit in his final at-bat (a notion known as the "gambler's fallacy"), any more than the chances are better than 50-50 of tossing tails after you've gotten heads several times in a row.

People with a lot of book smarts are prone to statistical muddleheadedness as well. Consider the following "guessing game" psychologist Eldar Shafir presented to 40 Princeton undergrads:

Under the black cover, each of the boxes is equally likely to be either white, blue, or purple. You are now offered to play one of the following two games of chance:

Game 1: You guess the color of the left-hand box. You win $5 if you were right, and nothing if you were wrong.

Game 2: You choose to uncover both boxes. You win $5 if they are the same color, and nothing if they are different colors.

Which game would you play? If you think about it for a moment, you'll see that in Game 1, the chances of guessing the color of one box are 1 in 3. In Game 2, whatever the color of the first box you uncover, the second box has to match it; in effect, the first box plays the role you do in game 1, of "guessing" the color of the other box. Again, you can see the chances are 1 in 3.

70% of the Princeton students, however, indicated a preference for Game 1, even though the chances of winning in each game are exactly the same. Why? Perhaps they wrongly assumed that in Game 2 they had to guess the color of both boxes rather than just one, which would indeed have lowered the odds. Maybe their problem-solving approach to Game 2 was influenced by the procedure for Game 1 (something psychologists call *perseveration*). The lesson? If you don't pay attention to the details of the problem, in both content and wording, you can't count on getting the right answer.

Think you're smarter than that? Try the logic problems in this section and see for yourself. In addition to the logical pitfalls described above, there's another you might want to keep an eye out for. Just because one particular answer seems more *representative* of the class of possible answers, that doesn't make it more *likely*. For example: If you were buying a lottery ticket, would you feel more confident selecting the sequence *1-1-1-1-1* or *1-11-18-25-39*? Most people would opt for the latter, since it seems more representative of the sorts of possible number sequences generated by a random process. In short, it seems more random. But that *doesn't* make it more likely. In fact, no single sequence of numbers is any more or less likely to win in any given drawing than any other — a fact which seems obvious once you think of it. Of course, the flip side of this is that if you're in the business of predicting *human* behavior, pure probability and statistics won't get you very far.

A final observation: If these probability problems give you a headache, keep in mind that they're good practice. Pushing an intuitively obvious idea to its logical conclusion may lead to a counterintuitive idea that is interesting and valuable precisely because nobody would have thought of it based on intuition alone. (A fundamental principle of information theory, after all, goes like this: "The importance of information is directly proportional to its improbability" — but here, "probability" means what *humans* think is probable, not what the *numbers* tell you is probable.) And training your mind to think in the cold, hard terms of mathematical probability may come in handy when you're considering placing a bet, either literally or figuratively, on some predicted outcome or other. Good luck!

At Barbara Bush High School in Ardmore, Oklahoma, 10th graders have the option of choosing either a home economics class or a shop class. There are three classes offered in each category: cake decorating, gardening, and interior design in home economics, and woodworking, auto mechanics, and computer repair in shop. Boys are a minority (45%) in the home economics category, and a majority (65%) in the shop category.

You enter a class at random, and you see that 55% of the students are boys. If you had to guess, which of the following would you choose:

1) It's probably a home economics class.
2) It's probably a shop class.
3) The chances are about even that it's home economics or shop.

BRAIN BITES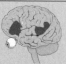

A variety of studies have shown how hormone levels might influence the stereotypical "female" skills (such as language, predominantly located in the left hemisphere), and "male" skills (such spatial skills as maze-running and imagining what an object might look like from a different angle, which are normally controlled in the right hemisphere). Psychologist Doreen Kimura at the University of Western Ontario reports that women's performance on verbal tasks peaks at the middle of their menstrual cycle, when the "female" hormones estrogen and progesterone are highest. Their spatial abilities, on the other hand, peak when their estrogen and progesterone are lowest. For men, testosterone appears to boost spatial intelligence, but only up to a point. E. Hampson has found that girls exposed to high levels of "male" hormones in the womb tend to have higher spatial intelligence. Hampson and S. D. Moffat have also shown, however, that men's performance on spatial tasks is worst in the morning, when testosterone is highest. Men's spatial performance rises later in the day, and in the springtime, when testosterone levels drop.

HINT: Don't be distracted by the fact that boys are a majority in this class.

I n the Mexican city of Oaxaca, the local public health department took a survey of all families with six children. In 72 families, the order of births (G = girls, B = boys) was GBBGBG.

Based on the information on the facing page, in about how
many families do you think the exact order of births was
GBGGGG?

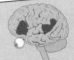

BRAIN BITES

British psychiatrist Stuart Dimond and German scientist Werner
Wittling have found, in separate studies, that a person's emotional response to movies will vary depending on which visual field
they're shown in. Dimond equipped the people in his experiment with a special contact lens that blocked out one-half of
their visual field. When only their left hemisphere was exposed
they responded more strongly to movies with a positive theme.
When they viewed movies with their right hemisphere, they
responded more strongly to movies with negative themes.
Wittling showed that movies viewed in the left visual field (link-
ing to the right brain) evoke a stronger stress response than
when shown in the right field (left brain). A study by researchers
Regard and Landis showed a similar effect with still pictures:
those shown to the left visual field (right brain) were disliked,
while those shown to the right field (left brain) were liked.

HINT: Don't confuse representativeness with probability.
Remember the lottery example.

In a small tribe in the highlands of New Guinea, there's a chief who allocates food rations to each of the tribe's five families. Each day, there are 20 yams to be handed out from the tribe's storehouse. Of course, the fair thing to do would be to distribute the yams evenly, according to the size of each family, but that's not how the chief likes to do it. Instead, he distributes 20 yams completely randomly each day. Sometimes, just by chance, the yams are handed out evenly among the families, but other times just one family may get all the yams, or one may get none. This way, the chief figures, the heads of the families will be more likely to bribe him with special favors, in an attempt to influence his decisions. But he's never influenced by the bribes at all. The absolute randomness of his allocations, he also figures, will nudge him towards the status of a deity in the tribe's eyes, since it's very hard for humans to be truly random in their choices.

Listed below are the allocations to the five families on two given days. The question: Over the course of a five years, will there be more days that match Monday's allocation, or Tuesday's allocation? Or will they end up being equally common?

Family	Monday	Tuesday
Atuanga	4	4
Biliki	3	4
Cicoro	5	4
Daru	4	4
Egats	4	4

BRAIN BITES

Left-brain verbal intelligence tests that require you to identify a connection between different things (for example, *orange* and *banana*, or *praise and punishment*) are called *similarities* tests. L. F. Jarvik points out that performance on similarities tests drops sharply between ages 75 and 86, even in test-takers with no signs of dementia.

HINT: There's a difference between this problem and a problem of the "lottery" type. Unlike in a lottery, it's not the case that each number's value is completely independent of the values of the others. If the first number in this series were 20, for example, then you can see in an instant that the four other numbers would be determined by that first choice.

PROBLEMATICS 4

Dr. Shapiro is the host of a popular late-night radio talk show that airs every night at 1 AM. His pet peeve is "fake" science — astrology, ESP, and the like. At the beginning of every show, to debunk the notion of telepathy, he selects a randomly-generated group of five numbers between 1 and 20, and "telepaths" them to the listeners. By the end of the show, he tabulates the results of the guesses called in by the listeners.

After about a year of this, Dr. Shapiro begins to notice some discomfiting patterns. The listeners seem to be much better at guessing some of the number sequences than others. For example, these randomly-generated sequences were guessed by more listeners than chance alone would dictate: 1, 5, 8, 13, 17; 3, 8, 11, 12, 16; and 4, 7, 10, 13, 18. (Nobody at all, on the other hand, guessed 1, 2, 3, 19, 20.)

Can you think of a reason, besides telepathy, that might explain why some number groups were easier for people to guess than others — and help dissuade Dr. Shapiro from cancelling this popular feature of his show?

BRAIN BITES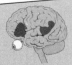

The neurological literature is replete with accounts of brain-damaged patients who develop bizarrely specific disorders. Vargha-Khadem, Isaacs and Mishkin report on a boy with a brain tumor who cannot remember anything he did that day. He can write it down, though, but not read what he writes. When someone else reads it back to him out loud, he's surprised by what he's written. When brain damage destroys reading ability but leaves writing skills intact, it's called *alexia without agraphia*. Norman Geschwind has explained this kind of syndrome as arising from damage to the connection between the right brain's visual processing regions and certain language processing areas in the left brain.

HINT: *To solve this one, you have to do the opposite of what the other puzzles require: Ask yourself why listeners would imagine the sequences indicated to be more likely than the one that nobody guessed.*

A pregnant mother in rural India, where boys are highly valued, wanted to do everything possible to increase her chances that her baby would be born a boy. She figured that some hospitals, for mysterious reasons, might have a better success rate, so to speak, at birthing boys than others. So she decided to find out which of two hospitals in her state had more days of the year on which at least 60% of the babies born were boys. The two hospitals were a small one in the town of Bandlapur about 100 miles from where she lived, and a much larger one only about 20 miles away. The large hospital performed many more deliveries overall, but there was a different statistic that was more important to her. She found to her delight that, indeed, one of the hospitals had 85 days of the year on which at least 60% of the babies born were boys, while the other hospital had only 20 such days.

Which hospital did she choose to go to for her delivery, the small one in Bandlapur or the larger one closer to home?

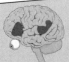

BRAIN BITES

If you think of an event from your past, do you see yourself in the memory as if you were an outsider looking at your younger self (*observer* mode), or do you look outward into the scene from your own younger eyes (*field* mode)? For memories from long ago, the answer is likely to be *observer*, for more recent memories *field*. Some psychologists believe that the field mode corresponds to an original memory, while the observer mode codes an indirect memory of a memory, mediated by the left brain's interpretive mechanism. Psychologists Nigro and Neisser have suggested that the mode may also depend on whether you're focusing on external circumstances or internal feelings. More recently, Robinson and Swanson have found that you can manipulate the emotional intensity of the memory by switching between the two modes.

HINT: As you know, the chances of giving birth to a boy or a girl are pretty much even. So then the question becomes: Would a large sample or a small one be more likely to reflect the overall even chances?

Here are a few of the unpleasant'st words
that ever blotted paper.

— William Shakespeare, *The Merchant of Venice* , Act III, circa 1597

ANASEARCHES

	B	A	N	G	L	E	S
				N			
				A			
E	L	B	A	T	O	P	
			O				
		R					

5 Word-Recognition
Short-Term
Memory Exercises

All about

ANASEARCHES

An Anasearch is a multi-part puzzle combining features of anagrams, crossword puzzles, and word searches. First, we'll give you a series of numbers which you translate into letters by the following rule: 1 = A, 2 = B, and so on. The result will be a word or (if there's a space in the number series) two words. For example: 14 1 2   12 5 7 would be NAB LEG.

Once you've written out the letters, you arrange those letters into a different word (or words) following a clue accompanying the numbers. For example: the clue "Bracelet" would lead you from NAB LEG to BANGLE. Some clues are clever, others (like the one just given) are more pedestrian. The tricky clues make reference to both the solution and the source. "Long-winded orator," for example, could get you from SNORE AT to SENATOR; "Drinkable to a *Polonais*" could get you from POLE TAB to POTABLE.

Next, you fill in an accompanying numbered grid by the same principle you used for the original translation of the number series into letters: 1 = A, etc. The final step is to find and circle the solved anagrams in the grid.

If you like anagrams but don't like word searches, you can just ignore the grid. If you want to make the puzzle harder, skip the first step of translating the numbers into letters. That way, all you'll have is a clue with nothing but the number of letters to help you get the solution (kind of like a crossword puzzle without any help from intersecting answers).

You can also ignore the clues in solving the anagrams — but you should always check your answer against the clue, since many of the anagrams have multiple possible solutions. For example,

SEE GRANT could be rearranged into either SERGEANT or ESTRANGE; the clue "Reason to part" tells you the latter is correct.

The many steps in an Anasearch puzzle draw on many different brain skills. The initial step of translating numbers into letters taxes your short-term or working memory (barring, at least, the unlikely event that you've already memorized the ordinal placement of every single letter of the alphabet). If the first item is 2 5 20, for example, you may automatically know that 2 = B, but most people will have to count from the beginning of the alphabet to figure out that 5 = E. Almost everyone has to count from A to get a letter value for 20 (which is T).

If the next line has 3 1 18, you can deduce the letter value for 18 either by counting from A all over again (the simple-minded approach), or you can count two letters backwards from T to get R — which taxes your attention, concentration, or what psychologists call *mental tracking* abilities. And if, a few lines down, 20 re-appears, you can either count from A again, or look back at the first line to remind yourself of the letter value, or try to remember the letter value from a few lines back. The first approach is simple-minded and time-consuming, the second is quicker but dependent on a crutch, while the third taxes your short-term memory and — if you remember well — can be quicker than looking back. By the time you get to the end of the puzzle, you probably will have memorized at least some number-letter correspondences you didn't already know.

The parts of your brain you'll be using are likewise numerous. As with the other letter- and word-manipulation puzzles in this book (Analocks, Alphabetics, etc.), you'll be using word-retrieval and semantic interpretation regions of your left hemisphere (Broca's and Wernicke's areas, for example). The added task of devising a quick and efficient system for translating numbers into their corresponding letters will tax "executive-attention" and planning regions of your frontal lobes, including areas to the front of Broca's. Recent PET scan studies show particularly strong activation of the left frontal lobe when verbal exercises impose a heavy burden on your working memory.

The less you rely on the crutch of looking back when you're translating the numbers into letters, the more you'll be using your working memory skills. Also, the less you look back, the more likely you'll end up memorizing at least some of the correspondences. If you were to do Anasearch puzzles regularly, repeated encounters with the number-values of all the letters of the alphabet would consolidate that knowledge into your long-term memory, which might come in handy for cryptic notes or party tricks.

19	12	5	14	4	5	18	5	19	20
12	20	22	17	21	5	5	11	18	5
1	13	9	19	1	12	20	5	4	18
16	1	12	16	5	7	1	19	21	19
19	18	19	5	5	20	9	18	3	5
20	9	14	19	19	14	14	19	3	1
9	14	14	20	14	14	4	14	15	20
3	5	15	5	8	5	1	1	5	20
11	18	20	18	14	18	5	5	12	12
20	19	5	19	20	21	13	2	12	5

Write out the letters corresponding to the numbers (A = 1, etc.), then rearrange the letters to make a new word fitting the clue provided. Finally, fill in each square in the grid (opposite) with its corresponding letter, and find and circle each of the answers in the grid. The first line is done for you.

Clues

A. 16 1 7 5 19   21 19   Winged horse (PAGES US, PEGASUS)
B. 19 12 9 3 11   16 1 19 20   Crude comedy
C. 19 16 5 14 4   9 20   Allowance
D. 18 5 9 14 13 1 18 19   While at sea, they dream of holding heavenly bodies
E. 12 1 19 20   20 5 5   Site of 18th hole in rainy locale
F. 12 5 14 4 19   20 18 5 5 19   Most willowy
G. 16 18 5 19 5 20 19   Teases
H. 14 5 1 18   9 20   Keep at hand
I. 2 5 12 20   19 21 13   A number do this in the boxing ring
J. 22 9 12 5   Very bad
K. 2 1 14 5 19   Bops in the noggin
L. 12 1 14 5 19   Tilts
M. 4 1 13 5   Honey wine
N. 19 14 9 20   British cans
O. 12 1 19 20 5 4   Preserved, in a way
P. 18 5 19 5 20   Succinct
Q. 20 9 18 5   One thing of Spring
R. 18 5 5 12   Ogle
S. 14 15 20 5   Famous English playing fields locale

BRAIN BITES

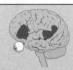

Brain researcher Robert Ornstein explains that, while it's the left hemisphere that's language-dominant for most people, it's the right brain that keeps track of many meanings simultaneously, as when you "get" a pun. Perhaps that's why people with right-brain strokes have a hard time with jokes.

HINT: D = MARINERS.

19	5	14	20	18	1	3	20	5	19
4	19	12	5	22	15	14	13	18	3
5	18	1	12	7	1	7	15	20	5
13	15	14	15	18	1	9	12	7	4
15	8	3	18	1	13	6	1	5	14
14	25	5	19	7	6	20	20	8	1
5	26	4	1	15	15	15	5	14	12
19	1	18	20	2	22	1	14	5	14
16	18	21	1	5	8	10	20	19	9
20	3	19	4	20	14	1	18	18	5

Write out the letters corresponding to the numbers (A = 1, etc.), then rearrange the letters to make a new word fitting the clue provided. Finally, fill in each square in the grid (opposite) with its corresponding letter, and find and circle each of the answers in the grid.

Clues

A. 2 15 1 20   1 7 5 19   Destruction by enemy agents
B. 20 5 5 14 19   3 1 18 20   High-brow intermission
C. 8 1 26 25   19 3 15 18 5 18   Little Big Horn victor
D. 3 8 1 18 13   Compelling music
E. 5 4   22 15 20 5 4   Ardent at election time
F. 18 1 14 20 5 18   A knight gone astray
G. 20 15   3 21 6 6   Interrupt (2 words)
H. 9 14 14   12 1 4   Not on the coast
I. 13 15 15 14   12 1 9 18   One way to a lunar den
J. 13 15 14 4 5   Not of this world
K. 20 1 12 5 14 20   Hidden
L. 14 1 22 5   Wind indicator
M. 19 12 15 22 5 14   Undisciplined short stories
N. 4 1 26 5   Axe relative
O. 3 12 5 1 14   Pierce with a sterile tool
P. 18 5 7 1 12   In the spotlight
Q. 7 15 1 20   Even a Greek one would not wear one

BRAIN BITES

A study by Zook and Dwyer concluded that levels of right-hemisphere abilities seem to develop equally across cultures regardless of educational opportunity, while development of the left hemisphere is more hampered by lack of education.

HINT: B = ENTR'ACTES.

ANASEARCH 3

14	18	15	13	21	18	20	19	15	14
8	9	25	1	23	5	20	1	7	18
19	16	19	12	15	19	21	19	18	5
4	18	14	3	5	15	20	20	5	20
1	15	5	7	15	18	21	9	14	19
13	1	1	20	15	20	18	16	9	5
14	23	4	16	18	15	14	4	13	23
5	24	16	5	10	15	9	14	1	9
4	1	24	9	15	13	16	5	24	14
18	5	23	1	18	4	19	19	5	7

Write out the letters corresponding to the numbers (A = 1, etc.), then rearrange the letters to make a new word fitting the clue provided. Finally, fill in each square in the grid (opposite) with its corresponding letter, and find and circle each of the answers in the grid.

Clues

A. 4 1 14 5 19   Sam ____, golfer

B. 20 15 14 9 3 19   Pick up a belle

C. 3 1 14 15 5   Not up the creek, in the ____, without a liner

D. 19 20 1 18 16 18 15 16   Harmonious relations

E. 19 20 9 16 5 14 4   To build a better cherry (2 words)

F. 13 1 4 4 5 14   What you become when you invoke God's wrath

G. 18 5 4 18 1 23   New effort pays off

H. 3 1 12 13   Silent, still

I. 7 5 20 1 23 1 25   Exit

J. 13 15 19 20 18 21 14   Some walk for a cure

K. 18 5 16 15 18 20 19   Bearers of tidings, or luggage

L. 19 23 1 7 5   Workers are dying for this

M. 19 16 21 18 20 9 14   Most don't rush for this food

N. 18 5 24 13 1 9 14 5   King of the dailies

O. 14 5 23 19 20 5 18   Occidental child

P. 24 - 20 18 5 5   Effort of former fir

Q. 23 5 19 9 14 7   Happy little women's work

R. 13 1 24 9 - 15   Largely self-evident truth

BRAIN BITES

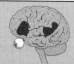

When the right hemisphere of the brain is temporarily paralyzed with sodium amytal, a short-acting anesthetic, the patient feels euphoric. When the left side of the brain is paralyzed, the patient feels tearful and depressed.

HINT: B = TOCSIN.

ANASEARCH 4

14	5	18	21	20	19	15	16	7	5
19	5	14	9	12	20	14	15	18	6
18	5	4	5	1	12	5	7	13	1
12	5	1	19	20	19	18	19	15	3
12	1	5	18	5	5	20	20	14	19
2	5	14	18	21	13	19	5	15	4
17	21	1	20	18	9	1	12	20	5
19	20	11	1	18	12	22	10	15	14
19	15	21	20	8	15	23	5	14	15
8	3	25	20	16	9	18	20	5	9

Write out the letters corresponding to the numbers (A = 1, etc.), then rearrange the letters to make a new word fitting the clue provided. Finally, fill in each square in the grid (opposite) with its corresponding letter, and find and circle each of the answers in the grid.

Clues

A. 19 20 15 18 5 21 16	Pose for the future
B. 12 9 14 5 14 6 18 15 19 20	Chilly trenches
C. 12 5 1 4 5 18	Double shuffle
D. 19 20 5 1 12	Take the littlest
E. 12 5 1 18	More tragic than fiction
F. 14 21 13 2 5 18	One relative of John Barleycorn (2 words).
G. 20 18 1 9 12	Test run
H. 12 1 18 11	A capital author
I. 20 15 23 14 8 15 21 19 5	Not North Owen (2 words)
J. 20 18 25 16 9 20 3 8	The three faces of Eve
K. 5 14 4 10 1 19 13 9 14 5	Where's Jim (3 words)?
L. 1 19 20 5 18	Gaze so hard you see stars
M. 5 7 15 19	For me, anything ___
N. 13 9 12 5 19	British scurvy medicine
O. 19 5 3 15 14 4	Single high mil. hon. (2 words)
P. 7 5 12 19 15 20	Start moving (2 words)
Q. 13 15 15 14 14 15 20 5	Dull sound
R. 6 1 3 5	Place for a pickup
S. 19 20 5 18 14	Nuts! (Slang)

BRAIN BITES

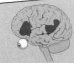

Language and basic musical skills are controlled by different parts of the brain. Even people who've lost all speech due to a left-hemisphere stroke may still be able to sing the words of a familiar song.

HINT: K = IN JAMES' DEN.

19	11	1	5	16	25	19	1	5	19
6	9	14	5	4	15	21	2	20	18
9	19	14	1	21	20	18	14	5	5
14	13	18	7	8	1	21	7	19	20
5	20	8	15	12	1	1	9	14	19
19	20	18	21	20	5	1	1	7	15
20	5	7	14	1	18	20	19	5	16
4	5	1	18	16	19	20	15	14	5
18	3	1	16	9	20	15	12	14	18
19	5	1	4	5	22	9	12	19	1

Write out the letters corresponding to the numbers (A = 1, etc.), then rearrange the letters to make a new word fitting the clue provided. Finally, fill in each square in the grid (opposite) with its corresponding letter, and find and circle each of the answers in the grid.

Clues

A. 20 9 14 7 12 5 19   15 14   Continuing pleasure in game of bridge

B. 19 16 5 1 11   25 5 1 19   Agree to bunny slopes (2 words)

C. 19 20 1 14 4   9 20   Put up with from afar

D. 6 5 4   9 14   2 15 21 20   Learn suspicion about boxing match
is justified (2 words)

E. 1 7 18 5 5   More than willing

F. 19 5 5   7 18 1 14 20   Reason to part

G. 9 5   18 1 16   19 1 16   In other words, rate maple syrup

H. 18 5 1 12   18 21 7   Is this floor covering special?

I. 4 1 18 20 19   Thrown for a violin

J. 16 18 5 19 20 15   A magic ad

K. 3 15 1 12   16 9 20   Building where there was a mine

L. 4 1 20 5   8 15 21 18   Wrote day and time

M. 1 21 14 20   19 20   Road named for a mocking relative

N. 20 18 21 19 20   A result of confidence

O. 9 14 6 5 19 20   It can happen to the best

P. 3 1 14 20 19   Hardly hypocritical

Q. 19 12 9 4 5   22 1 19 5   Water sprites play with urn (2 words)

R. 18 5 1 4   John, in a letter

S. 15 21 7 8 20 19   Had to look

T. 15 14 5   19 20   Monument on First Ave.

U. 1   18 15 16 5   Thereby hangs a tale

BRAIN BITES

Psycholinguists tell us that during the second through sixth years of life, children learn about ten new words a day. At age one and a half, the average child has a vocabulary of about 30-50 words; by age six, she's mastered at least 10,000.

HINT:
A = SINGLETON.

Nothing proves more clearly that the mind seeks truth, and nothing reflects more glory upon it, than the delight it takes, sometimes in spite of itself, in the driest and thorniest researches of algebra.

— Bernard de Fontenelle, in the preface to *Histoire du renouvellement de l'Académie des Sciences*, 1708

ALGEBRA
GAMES

5 Math-Rule Operations

$$5 \times 5 \div 5 + 5 = 10$$
$$5 \times 5 + (5 \div 5) = 26$$
$$5 \times [(5 \div 5) \times 5] = 25$$
$$5 - [(5 - 5) \times 5] = 5$$

All about

ALGEBRA GAMES

$$5 \times 5 \div 5 + 5 = 10$$
$$5 \times 5 + (5 \div 5) = 26$$
$$5 \times [(5 \div 5) \times 5] = 25$$
$$5 - [(5 - 5) \times 5] = 5$$

There's an old brain-teaser that goes like this. A professor gives his class a test with the following problem: Transform nine "hads" in a row ("had had had had had had had had had") into a proper sentence; words may be added before or after the series, and punctuation is permitted.

The answer: "In the examination John, where Jim had 'had', had 'had had'. 'Had had' had had the examiner's approval."

Algebra Games are very much like this word puzzle, except that the pieces of the puzzle are numbers and arithmetical signs like "=" and "x" rather than words and punctuation marks. For example:

$$2 \ 2 \ 2 = 2$$

If you want to make this equation true, you can fill in arithmetical signs like this:

$$2 + 2 - 2 = 2$$

or like this:

$$(2 + 2) \div 2 = 2$$

or this:

$$(2 \times 2) \div 2 = 2$$

As you can see, just as in the word puzzle, there are many possibilities that count as valid solutions — a fact which makes Algebra Games easier than they might otherwise be. Unlike some of the other types of puzzles in this book, you can do each line independently of the others, another feature that eases the cognitive burden on the puzzle solver.

The simplest Algebra Games involve the simplest operations, like addition or multiplication, performed in left-to-right linear sequence — as in the first solution on the previous page. More complex answers may involve more complex operations — like "the square root of" — or may yield a correct answer only if you perform the operations in a certain order. To see how the order of operations can affect the answer, consider how putting the parentheses in a different place changes the outcome of the second answer on the previous page:

$$2 + (2 \div 2) = 3$$

The simplest way to think of parentheses is that they require you to do everything inside them — in this case, dividing 2 by 2 — before performing the operations that are written outside them — in this case, addition.

Sometimes, to keep things straight, it helps to group parentheses within parentheses. By convention, for visual clarity, the outer parentheses are written as square brackets. For example, see if you can solve this one:

$$9\ 9\ 9\ 9 = 9$$

Two possible answers are as follows:

$$[(9 - 9) \times 9] + 9 = 9$$
$$9 - [(9 - 9) \times 9] = 9$$

Again, see what a difference it would make to group the numbers and signs in a different way:

$$(9 - 9 - 9) \times 9 = -81$$

Since we use square roots in some of our solutions, you need to remember that the square root of a given number is a number that, when multiplied by itself, yields that given number. For example, the square root of 4 is 2, of 9 is 3, of 16 is 4, etc. The symbol for square root is "$\sqrt{\ }$."

Want more practice? Try this one:

$$4 \ 4 \ 4 \ 4 = 15$$

Once again, there are multiple possible solutions. Here are two:

$$[4 \div (-4)] + (4 \times 4) = 15$$
$$(4 \times 4) - (4 \div 4) = 15$$

Now, try this one:

$$4 \ 4 \ 4 \ 4 = 16$$

Two answers are as follows:

$$(4 \times 4) \div (4 \div 4) = 16$$
$$\sqrt{4} \times \sqrt{4} \times \sqrt{4} \times \sqrt{4} = 16$$

On the other hand, a much simpler one is this:

$$4 + 4 + 4 + 4 = 16$$

If you missed the obvious solution, don't feel bad. Once your left hemisphere gets really proficient at applying some of the more complex analyses, you may overlook some easy ones. (The right hemisphere, by contrast, tends to approach any problem as if it's never encountered a similar one before.) Psychologists refer to this as an *Einstellung* effect, meaning that you get stuck in a particular mode of thinking. But while an *Einstellung* experience may make you feel silly, it's also evidence that you've been paying attention.

$$( ) \times - = 10$$
$$( ) \times \times + = 10$$
$$( ) \times \times + \div = 10$$
$$( ) \times + \div \sqrt{} = 10$$
$$+ = 10$$
$$[(+ \times) - (+)] \div = 10$$
$$[ ] ( ) ( ) \times + + + \div = 10$$
$$[ ] ( ) ( ) + + \times \div = 10$$
$$( ) \times + \div = 10$$

In this first Algebra Game puzzle, you're given both the numbers and the mathematical signs you'll need to get a correct answer. Combine arithmetical signs and and identical digits (not more than six digits in each equation) on each line as needed to express 10 as the answer to the equation you construct. Begin on the first line using only 1's. Continue on the second line using only 2's (hint: you'll need only four 2's) and so on through to the last line where you use only 9's. All the *plus*, *minus*, *times*, *divided by*, and *square root* signs are in an order you can use in the answer we figured out — except for line 8. (You'll still have to figure out where to put the parentheses and brackets; square brackets go around curved parentheses, as we've shown you in line 6.)

Starters: Eleven is made of two 1's next to each other. The only times we used up all six digits in an equation were on the line using 6's and the line using 7's. The square root of 4 is 2.

BRAIN BITES

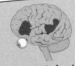

Prentice Starkey at the University of Pennsylvania and his colleague Robert G. Cooper designed a clever experiment to prove that even before an infant can count, he recognizes the difference between 1, 2, 3, and 4. In the experiment, Starkey and Cooper showed newborns a pattern of three dots. The infants were interested until the same number of dots was re-shown enough times that they became "habituated." Add or subtract a dot, however, and they immediately perked up again. (The newborns didn't have the ability to tell the difference between larger numbers of dots, such as six or seven.)

HINT: One possible answer for line 3 is "(3 × 3 × 3 + 3) ÷ 3 = 10."

$$7 \quad 7 \quad 7 \quad 7 \quad = \quad 1$$
$$7 \quad 7 \quad 7 \quad 7 \quad = \quad 2$$
$$7 \quad 7 \quad 7 \quad 7 \quad = \quad 3$$
$$7 \quad 7 \quad 7 \quad 7 \quad = \quad 6$$
$$7 \quad 7 \quad 7 \quad 7 \quad = \quad 8$$
$$7 \quad 7 \quad 7 \quad 7 \quad = \quad 13$$
$$7 \quad 7 \quad 7 \quad 7 \quad = \quad 15$$
$$7 \quad 7 \quad 7 \quad 7 \quad = \quad 48$$
$$7 \quad 7 \quad 7 \quad 7 \quad = \quad 49$$
$$7 \quad 7 \quad 7 \quad 7 \quad = \quad 56$$

Insert arithmetical signs between these numbers to make the equations true. The fewer signs you use, the better. These are the signs we used in our answer: *plus*, *minus*, *times*, *divided by*, *square root*, parentheses, and brackets. (Parentheses and square brackets serve the same function of grouping numbers and signs together; by convention, square brackets go outside parentheses, like this: [(2 x 2 -2) x 2] -2 = 2.)

BRAIN BITES

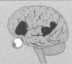

Along with superior verbal abilities, many studies show that women are better than men at detecting whether one item in a collection of small objects has been removed, and at detecting subtle differences among visually similar objects. Men tend to be slightly better at certain other right-brain spatial tasks. Why might we have evolved that way? If these differences developed, as many have assumed, during pre-agricultural hunter-gatherer times, then women's foraging role may have placed a premium on detecting small changes in a close environment. As primary nurturers, women would also have carried the burden of passing knowledge to infants and small children, a situation that may have selected for superior language abilities. If men were primarily hunters, navigational and orientational skills would have been important. Researchers such as S. J. Gaulin have also noted superior spatial abilities among the males of polygamous animal species, so the human pattern may point to a polygamous evolutionary history.

HINT: Our answer for the fifth line is "(7
$x\ 7) + [7 \div 7] = 8.$"

$$2 \quad 2 \quad 2 \quad 2 \quad = \quad 0$$
$$2 \quad 2 \quad 2 \quad 2 \quad = \quad 1$$
$$2 \quad 2 \quad 2 \quad 2 \quad = \quad 2$$
$$2 \quad 2 \quad 2 \quad 2 \quad = \quad 3$$
$$2 \quad 2 \quad 2 \quad 2 \quad = \quad 4$$
$$2 \quad 2 \quad 2 \quad 2 \quad = \quad 5$$
$$2 \quad 2 \quad 2 \quad 2 \quad = \quad 6$$
$$2 \quad 2 \quad 2 \quad 2 \quad = \quad 7$$
$$2 \quad 2 \quad 2 \quad 2 \quad = \quad 10$$
$$2 \quad 2 \quad 2 \quad 2 \quad = \quad 12$$

Insert arithmetical signs between these numbers to make the equations true. The fewer signs you use, the better. These are the signs we used in our answer: *plus, minus, times, divided by*, parentheses, and brackets. (Parentheses and square brackets serve the same function of grouping numbers and signs together; by convention, square brackets go outside parentheses, like this: [(2 x 2 -2) x 2] -2 = 2.)

Starters: In our answer for the "7" line, we placed a decimal point before the second 2.

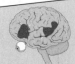

BRAIN BITES

Gray matter in the brain makes up the cerebral cortex, the "thinking cap" on the surface of the brain containing the bodies and dendrites of brain cells, while the white matter beneath consists of axons forming long-distance connections between the brain cells. University of Pennsylvania neurobiologist Ruben Gur and colleagues have determined that the right hemisphere has a higher ratio of "white matter" to "gray matter" than the left. When Stuart Dimond and D. Blizard analyzed the right hemisphere they found it also had more total tissue than the left. Elkhonon Goldberg and Louis Costa have interpreted the foregoing research findings to mean that the right hemisphere is built to integrate data from widely-scattered sites of the cortex, while the left is designed to handle discrete packets of information in efficient, modular fashion.

HINT: Our answer for the "7" line is "[(2 ÷ .2) ÷ 2] + 2 = 7."

$$3 \quad 3 \quad 3 \quad 3 \quad = \quad 3$$

$$3 \quad 3 \quad 3 \quad 3 \quad = \quad 4$$

$$3 \quad 3 \quad 3 \quad 3 \quad = \quad 5$$

$$3 \quad 3 \quad 3 \quad 3 \quad = \quad 6$$

$$3 \quad 3 \quad 3 \quad 3 \quad = \quad 7$$

$$3 \quad 3 \quad 3 \quad 3 \quad = \quad 8$$

$$3 \quad 3 \quad 3 \quad 3 \quad = \quad 9$$

$$3 \quad 3 \quad 3 \quad 3 \quad = \quad 10$$

Insert arithmetical signs between, before, and after the 3's to produce the numbers 1 through 10. In our answer, we used these signs: *plus*, *minus*, *times*, *divided by*, parentheses, and brackets.

B R A I N   B I T E S

Idiot savants are people who combine a phenomenal skill — say, a photographic memory for music or for trivial facts such as license plate numbers — with subnormal intelligence in other domains. One theory, proposed by psychologist Terry L. Brink, holds that they may get this way from some kind of left-brain damage, which forces their right hemisphere to become unusually strong in compensation. (Albert Einstein, too, displayed much stronger right-brain than left-brain skills; his powers of visual thinking were phenomenal, but his left-brain language abilities were relatively weak. His fame as a theoretical physicist came from his powers of visualization, not skill in manipulating numbers.)

HINT: Our answer for the third line is "$(3 + 3) - (3 \div 3) = 5$."

4   4   4   4   =   1
4   4   4   4   =   2
4   4   4   4   =   3
4   4   4   4   =   4
4   4   4   4   =   5
4   4   4   4   =   6
4   4   4   4   =   7
4   4   4   4   =   8
4   4   4   4   =   9
4   4   4   4   =   10

Insert arithmetical signs between, before, and after the 4's to produce the numbers 1 through 10. In our answer, we used these signs: *plus*, *minus*, *times*, *divided by*, *square root*, parentheses, and brackets.

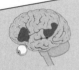

BRAIN BITES

The influential "right-shift" theory of Marion Annett of the University of Hull in England offers a genetic explanation for handedness. A dominant gene codes for speech in the left hemisphere, increasing the chances of right-handed manual skill. A recessive version of the gene results in no innate left or right preference for speech or handedness. That means that if you inherit the recessive version from both your mother and your father (which would occur in about 25% of the population), you'll be about equally likely to end up left- or right-handed. Cultural factors might result in a little over half of this group being right-handed. If you do the math, you'll see this model correctly predicts that only about 10% of people will be left-handed.

HINT: Our answer for the fourth line is "(4 x 4) ÷ (√4 + √4) = 4."

If we condemn natural magic, or the wisdom of nature, because the Devil (who knoweth more than any man) doth also teach witches and poisoners the harmful parts of herbs, drugs, minerals and excrements, then we may by the same rule condemn the physician and the art of healing.

— Sir Walter Raleigh, *History of the World,* VOL I, 1614

The magician is an infidel, but his magic is truth — A Hindu proverb

MAGIC SQUARES

5 Number-Logic Concentration Exercises

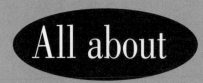
All about

MAGIC
SQUARES

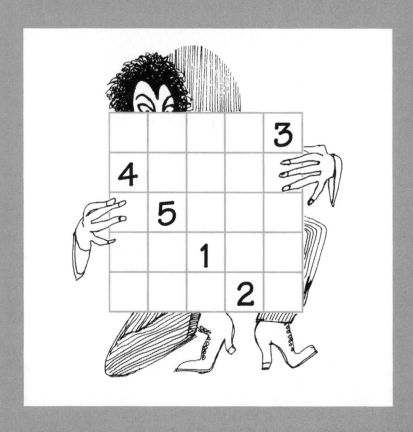

The "magic" in the name of this puzzle category isn't the invention of some latter-day puzzle promoter. For thousands of years, in ancient civilizations as far-flung as Babylonia, India, China, and Greece, Magic Squares have been held to have mystical significance.

The basic idea of a Magic Square is simple enough. A Magic Square is a grid of numbers that add up to a given total in any direction, horizontal, vertical, or diagonal; each number must be different from all the others in the grid. The simplest possible Magic Square, apart from a single number, is a 3 x 3 grid (a 2 x 2 Magic Square is impossible to construct):

If you add three numbers in any direction in this grid, you'll see they always add up to 15.

So far, so good. Intriguingly enough, though, there's only one possible arrangement of the numbers 1-9 (apart from merely rotating the entire square) that will result in a Magic Square. The grid has another interesting feature: the sum of any two numbers on opposite sides of the center number (e.g., 6 + 4, 3 + 7, etc.) always equals the sum of the first and last numbers in the series (1 and 9). The question of whether patterns like this might be more than mere coincidence has always contributed to the aura of mystery and magic surrounding Magic Squares.

If you want to construct a Magic Square of your own, there's a simple recipe to follow. (This works only for odd-number Magic Squares, like grids of 3 x 3, 5 x 5, etc., not even-number ones.) If you imagine a Magic Square circling back on itself in a certain way (see next page), then all you have to do is start in the top center square and, always moving one square up and to the right, place consecutive numbers in each adjacent diagonal square. After moving three squares for a 3 x 3 grid (5 for a 5 x 5, etc.), drop one square down and continue writing consecutive numbers diagonally.

Why does this procedure result in a Magic Square? You're free to speculate. There are many other odd-number Magic Squares that don't fit this pattern (so Magic Square afficionados need never get

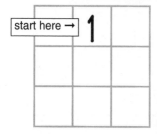

bored), and other Magic Square construction techniques that work just as well, but the procedure just described always works. (There's an equally reliable, but completely different, procedure for creating an even-number Magic Square.)

"Magic" shapes other than squares can be constructed, too. Some of the most popular ones are Magic Cubes, Magic Stars, Magic Hexagons, and Magic Triangles. Each has its own particular rules, but the basic idea remains the same: the numbers must all add up to the same total in any direction. (There are also "antimagic" squares, with the numbers arranged so that they never add up to the same total in any direction.)

In general, the more dimensions and intersections the shape has, the harder it is to fill in numbers to fit a "magic" pattern. Three-dimensional Magic Cubes are much harder to solve than two-dimensional Magic Squares, and four-sided Magic Squares are harder to solve than equivalently-sized three-sided Magic Triangles. You can see in an instant why this should be if you try your hand at solving a Magic X, which contains only a single intersection. Given the numbers 1-5, fit them into squares in the X below such that they add up to the same total in either diagonal direction:

If you follow the common-sense strategy of placing in the center of the X the number that is mid-way between the two extremes (1 and 5), then you'll start with the 3 in the center position. From there, you can readily see that you'll want to avoid lining up

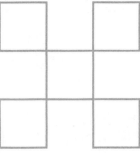

the two highest numbers or the two lowest ones in the same row. So you balance the highest (5) with the lowest (1), and place the 2 and 3 on the other branch of the X. The result is a simple Magic X with each diagonal row adding up to 9:

The strategy of placing a "middle" number in a "middle" position is one that will serve you well in many "magic" puzzles. The principle of balancing a high number with a low one also often comes in handy. We'll give you other tips in the instructions for each puzzle.

Since "magic" shapes with the complexity of a square or greater can be vexingly difficult even for the most die-hard number puzzle nut, we've included mostly Magic Triangles and smaller, simpler variants of the Magic Square format in this selection.

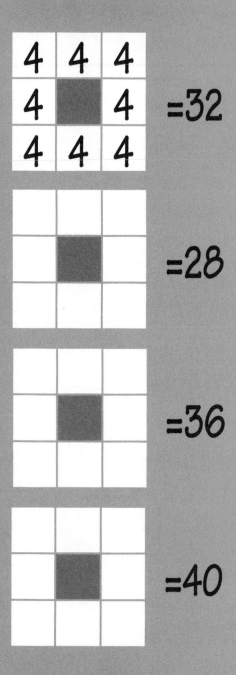

This variation on the Magic Square theme involves only horizontal and vertical dimensions, and you're allowed to use numbers more than once in a grid.

The numbers in the top grid add up to 32. Each horizontal row and vertical column adds up to 12. Can you make three additional squares with total values of 28, 36, and 40? You must make each row and column add up to 12 while alternating different digits in each square.

Starters: Placing larger numbers in the corners results in a smaller total since each corner number contributes twice to row/column totals but only once to the overall total.

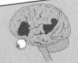

BRAIN BITES

Even though the right hemisphere is often characterized as having more "spatial" skills than the left, neuroimaging studies show that there are many spatial tasks for which the left dominates. Familiar objects and visual patterns, including familiar faces, are often processed in the left brain. Less routine visual or spatial tasks, including maze-running and imagining what an object would look like from a different perspective, are more right-brain-dependent. That's why neuroscientists Sally Springer and Georg Deutsch, from the University of California at Davis and the University of Alabama respectively, refer to the right hemisphere's skills as *manipulospatial*.

HINT: Place a 5 in each corner of the "28" square.

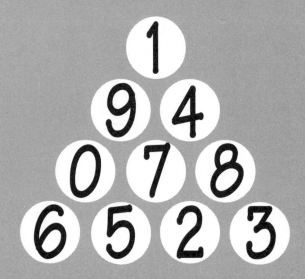

The digits 0 through 9, shown in the figure to the left, add up to 16 on each side of the triangle. Rearrange them for another, smaller number. More than one solution is possible.

Starters: Since only the numbers on the edges count towards the total (16 in the example given), you can "deactivate" any of the 10 numbers in the triangle by moving it to the center. If you want to get a smaller total than the 16 in the example at left, you should take one of the numbers larger than 7 and move it to the center.

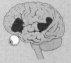

BRAIN BITES

S. Coren of the University of British Columbia reports the results of a study showing that left-handed men show higher *divergent thinking* scores than right-handed men. Divergent thinking differs from the *convergent thinking* measured by traditional intelligence tests in that divergent thinking tests measure the quantity and variety of answers, rather than simply the ability to come up with a single "correct" answer. ("What are the possible uses of a brick?" would be a typical divergent thinking question.) Coren speculates that divergent reasoning ability may be linked to the right hemisphere, which some researchers have argued to be more dominant among left-handers than right-handers.

HINT: *Start by moving the largest number to the center, and the smallest numbers to the corners.*

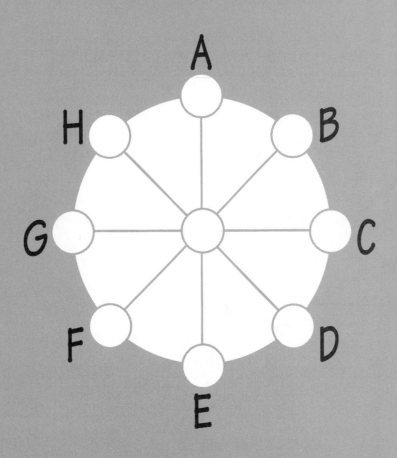

52 56 60 64 68 72 76 80 84

Place each of the numbers listed below the Magic Number-Ring so that:

1. The three numbers on each straight line equal 204.
2. The numbers in arcs ABC, CDE, EFG, and GHA also equal 204.

Starters: A systematic, linear approach to this puzzle would be to first list all the three-number combinations from the list that add up to 204. The number that occurs most frequently in these combinations will go in the middle, and the next most frequently-occurring ones will go at the ends of each of the arcs.

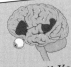

BRAIN BITES

A recent PET scan study by Toronto researcher Shitij Kapur and colleagues confirmed that, if you want to memorize a list of words, *semantic* coding (e.g., judging whether a noun represents a living or nonliving thing) works better than shallow *perceptual* coding (e.g., checking for the letter *a* in each noun). The PET scans showed that it was the front part of the left hemisphere (left inferior frontal cortex) that was active during the semantic coding task.

HINT: The number halfway through the list, 68, will also go in the center of the Magic Number-Ring.

MAGIC SQUARE 4

			4
	3		
		2	
1			

The numbers 1, 2, 3, and 4 have been strategically positioned in the opposite grid to permit the construction of Magic Square. By correctly placing each of the numbers 5 through 16 in the remaining blank boxes, the sum of the numbers in the boxes will be the same when added horizontally, vertically, and diagonally. In this case, the magic number is 34.

Starters: The numbers in the two blank inside boxes total 29. The numbers in the two blank corner boxes also total 29.

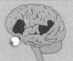

BRAIN BITES

Rear right-brain strokes often cause "constructional" problems, with a patient unable to assemble pieces into a coherent whole, or problems following directions or finding one's way around. But right-brain damage can also lead to *spatial dyscalculia*, difficulty performing mathematical calculations. The two kinds of problem are linked: since the patient has problems processing visual information, he may neglect the left side of a column of numbers, or "carry" decimal places incorrectly. Mathematical concepts, however, are unaffected, as is the ability to perform mathematical operations in one's head.

HINT: The number in the top left corner is 15; the number in the bottom right corner is 14.

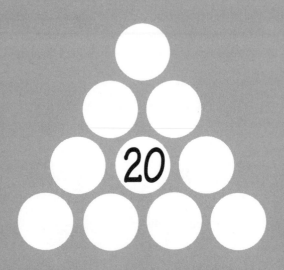

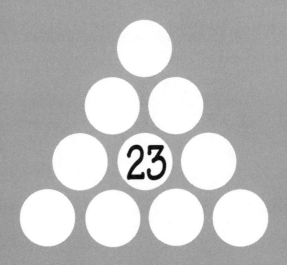

An equilateral triangle has all legs equal. By placing the digits 1 through 9 properly, the two identical triangles to the left can be arithmetically equilateral. But in one the digits placed in the circles on each of the sides will total 20; in the other triangle, each side will total 23.

BRAIN BITES

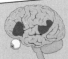

We all know that the right side of the brain keeps track of what is happening on the left side of the body, and vice versa. And, for most of us, only the left side of our brain is able to *talk* about what's going on anywhere. So, what happens if the right side of the brain can no longer send information to the left side so it can describe what is going on there? Some epilepsy patients have bene- fitted from an operation that severs the connection between the two halves of the brain. After the operation, neither side can send information to the other. In all obvious respects, people who have had that operation seem to behave just like you and me. Why? Partly because the "verbal" left hemisphere can still use indirect evidence to deduce what the right brain is experiencing, much as a driver can figure out that an obscured traffic light must be red or green by the way the other cars are moving. For example, if a split- brain patient thrusts his left hand into his pocket and feels a comb, the right side of his brain knows it is a comb, but it cannot com- municate that fact to the left hemisphere. The puzzle is that the patient can often still say that there's a comb in his left pocket. How does he do it? Careful observation reveals that he quickly and automatically rubs his fingers along the comb's teeth as soon as he feels it — which allows the left brain to pick up on the identity of the object by the *sound* it makes.

But that I am forbid to tell the secrets of my prison-house, I could a tale unfold whose slightest word would harrow up thy soul .

— William Shakespeare, *Hamlet,* Act I, circa 1600

CODEBREAKERS

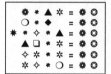

5 Deductive Symbol-to-Math
Encryptions

All about

CODEBREAKERS

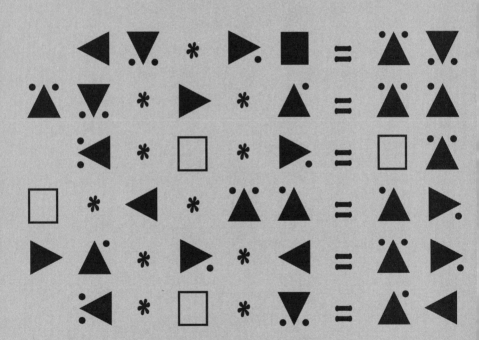

Codebreakers are one of the hardest puzzle types in this book, but also one of the most satisfying to solve. The puzzles require you to do essentially what a military decoding expert does: translate encrypted information into an understandable message.

In our Codebreakers, you'll find rows of strange-looking symbols that you'll have to translate into numbers and, sometimes, into mathematical signs like "+" and "-". The goal is to end up with an equation that makes mathematical sense. For example: ✵ + ❀ = ♥.

For this line, many answers are possible. ✵ could equal, say, 3, ❀ could equal 4, and ♥ could equal 7. But let's say the next line was as follows: ✵ X ❀ = ♣.

Once you see this second line, you know immediately that the values we just gave the first two symbols must be wrong, since 3 x 4 would be 12, a two-digit number, while there's only a single symbol to the right of the equals sign. So you know that whatever ✵ and ❀ are, they must equal 9 or less when multiplied together. You know that neither symbol could be 0, since otherwise on the first line one of the symbols would reappear to the right of the equals sign — any number plus 0 equals that same number. (The second line rules out 0 as well; we'll let you figure out why.) The second line also rules out 1 for a value for either symbol, since any number times 1 equals that same number, so one of the symbols to the left of the equals sign would reappear to the right.

So the two symbols could be 2 and 4, or 2 and 3, or 4 and 2, or 3 and 2. But which of the four possibilities *are* they? The third line solves it: ♣ - ✵ = ✵.

This, along with the other two lines, helps you to single out 4 as the value for ❋, and therefore 2 as the value for ❀, and therefore 6 as the value for ♥ and 8 as the value for ♣.

In walking you through the example here, we've shown you some of the most basic rules that all Codebreaker puzzles share. A symbol may be any positive digit from 0 to 9. A single symbol is always a one-digit number. Two symbols together are a two-digit number. Any given symbol always has the same value within a puzzle, wherever it appears.

You've also gotten a sense of the principles that make Codebreakers such intriguing puzzles to solve. Almost any single line in isolation has multiple solutions. But taken together, all the lines permit only one single number-value for each symbol. The puzzle as a whole forms a delicately and perfectly interlocking structure; substitute a single incorrect value in any line and the whole structure collapses like a house of cards.

Both the interdependency of the lines and values and the fact that almost any line in isolation could mean any of a number of things make solving a Codebreaker similar to learning a language. When you think of what an infant has to go through in order to decipher the curious noises around her, it's remarkable that language acquisition takes place at all. Unlike you or me, she can't figure out what some words mean by making reference to other words, the way we might learn the meaning of a new word like *meretricious* with reference to familiar ones like "alluring by false, showy charms." After all, you can't decipher meaningless sounds by translating them into other meaningless sounds. What the infant has to do is begin with something relatively easy, like associating the word *duckie* with a little yellow object she can see. Bit by bit, and with the help of innate rules and principles (much like the knowledge of logic and algebra, and of a general understanding of the rules of the puzzle, that you bring to the task of solving a Codebreaker), she can build on the easier elements and bootstrap her way up to more complex locutions.

The Codebreakers that can really get difficult are the ones where you have to figure out mathematical signs in addition to numbers — in other words, where we don't even tell you whether you should add, subtract, multiply or divide the numbers together: ❄ * ●● = ❄❄.

If all you know is that the * is some mathematical sign or other, but you don't know which, it might seem an impossible task to begin to pin down a single value for any of the symbols. So how do you do it? Essentially, by the same principles applied to the easier examples, along with a little help we'll give you. Let's say we tell you that the value of the ❄ is 3. Even without this hint, you could rule out *minus* or *divided by* for the value of the mathematical sign, for obvious reasons. And you could even rule out *plus*, as you can immediately see by trying any number-values at random for the two symbols ❄ and ●. So that leaves only *times*, and the ● must be 1, and so even without our help you can see how you can start to figure out some of the symbols' values even when none are given. With the hint, you can solve the line as follows: 3 x 11 = 33.

Then, let's say the next line is as follows: ● ✲ * ❄ = ▲.

Right away, you can rule out *plus* or *times* for the mathematical sign, and you can begin to narrow down possibilities for the other symbols. Further lines will help rule out some of those possibilities, and by the time you get to the end, using other lines to narrow down multiple possibilities as you progress, you'll have solved the puzzle.

Codebreaker 1

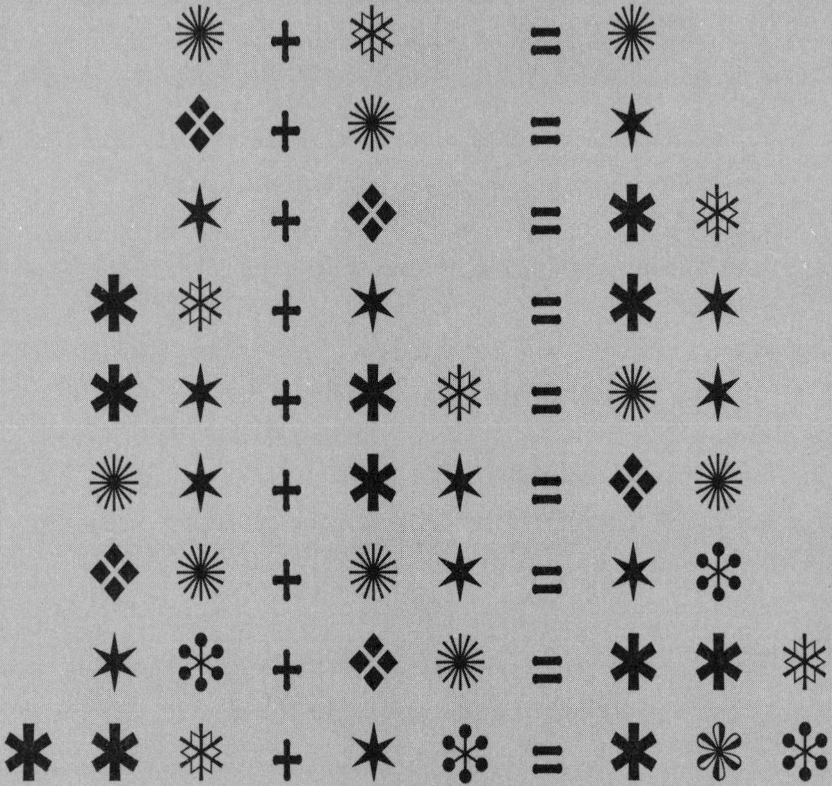

The "Starters" paragraphs and "Hints" (printed upside down) for many puzzles will help you get started again if you are stuck. However, all the puzzles are solvable without them. If you want to make the puzzles more challenging, just ignore those clues.

Each symbol, as it is used in this puzzle, represents a digit, always the same digit. Here's some help on strategy: The first line tells you the value of ✳. The third line tells you the value of ✱, and helps you begin to narrow down the values of the symbols on the left of the equation.

Starters: ❖ = 4, ✳ = 2, and ✱ = 6.

BRAIN BITES

If it's true that the specific respective strengths of the left and right hemispheres reflect fundamentally different modes of thought or data processing, then perhaps our brain evolved hemispheric asymmetry because the different modes might interfere with each other if they were located together in the same hemisphere. So argues cognitive scientist Jerre Levy.

HINT: The solution to the third line from the end is "42 + 26 = 68."

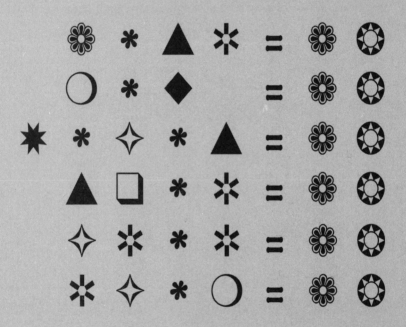

Each symbol represents a digit, always the same digit. The asterisk represents a mathematical sign, but not necessarily the same sign in each equation.

Starters: ✳ = 2 and ✿ = 3.

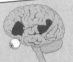

BRAIN BITES

Damage to one side of the brain can cause a phenomenon called *neglect*. If your right hemisphere is damaged in the areas that process vision, you may be unaware of seeing anything in your left visual field (which links to the right hemisphere). Your eyes would be working just fine, and they would be sending all the proper input to your primary visual areas in your occipital lobes, but your brain wouldn't be processing the input properly "downstream" from there. So the information would be getting into your brain, but you wouldn't be consciously aware of it. For some reason, damage to the left brain's visual areas rarely results in neglect.

HINT: The solution to line 1 is "3 x 12 = 36."

CODEBREAKER 3

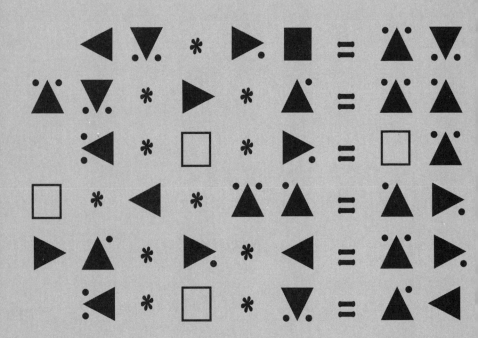

Each symbol represents a digit, always the same digit. The asterisk represents a mathematical sign, but not necessarily the same sign in each equation. Here are some strategy suggestions: The values you're given for the first line help you narrow down the possibilities for the unfilled values on that line. Line 2 helps you finish solving line 1, and line 3 helps confirm your answer.

Starters: □ = 9, ■ = 0, ◤= 1, ▼.= 2, ◣ = 3, and ▲ = 5.

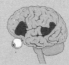

BRAIN BITES

The brain hemisphere that's more active will use more blood. So your ear temperature on that side of your head will be lower. On the other hand, Australian neuroscientist Jack Pettigrew has found that pouring ice water into one ear will activate the opposite side of the brain. (Don't try this at home — professional medical supervision is advised.)

HINT: The solution for the second line is "12 + 6 - 3 = 15."

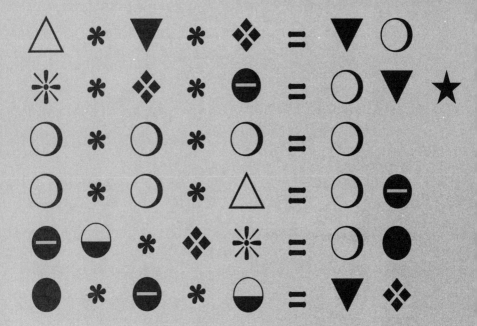

Each symbol represents a digit, always the same digit. The asterisk represents a mathematical sign, but not necessarily the same sign in each equation. Lines 1, 4, 5, and 6 form a useful interlocking group: they help you to rule out ambiguous values for symbols on other lines.

Starters: ▼ = 2, ● = 3, and ○ = 1.

HINT: The answer to the second line is "4 x 5 x 6 = 120."

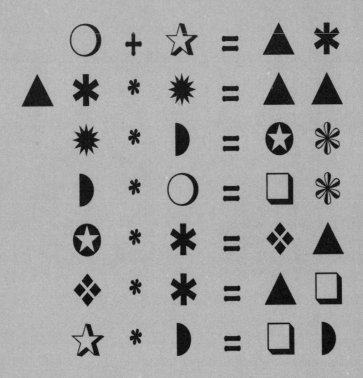

Each symbol represents a digit, always the same digit. The asterisk represents a mathematical sign, but not necessarily the same sign in each equation. The addition sign on the first line gives you a leg-up. Strategy help: Line 1 will point you to the number value of ▲ ; once you have this, you can deduce the value of the mathematical sign in line 5, and go on from there.

Starters: ❋ = 0 and ✱ = 7.

BRAIN BITES

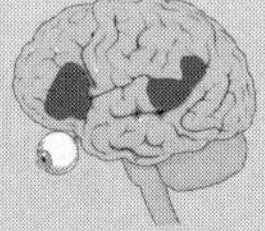

Brain researchers Norman Geschwind and Albert Galaburda have proposed a hormonal theory of handedness. Elevated testosterone in the womb slows the development of the fetus's left hemisphere, with the right hemisphere developing correspondingly more rapidly. Both male and female fetuses are exposed to testosterone, but males more than females. So more boys will be left-handed and have superior right-hemisphere skills, such as spatial intelligence. Since testosterone may also harm the immune system, more boys and left-handers in general will have immune disorders such as allergies and asthma.

HINT: The solution to line 1 is "8 + 9 = 17."

ANALOCKS

Analock Intro — page 22

T	H	R	O	W
H	E	A	V	E
R	A	Y	O	N
O	V	O	I	D
W	E	N	D	S

Analock #1 — page 24

S	H	A	V	E
H	A	V	E	N
A	V	E	R	T
V	E	R	S	E
E	N	T	E	R

Analock #2 — page 26

V	I	S	I	T
I	R	I	S	H
S	I	L	L	Y
I	S	L	A	M
T	H	Y	M	E

Analock #3 — page 28

S	T	A	R	T
T	A	B	O	R
A	B	O	D	E
R	O	D	I	N
T	R	E	N	D

Analock #4 — page 30

P	L	A	T	A
L	E	G	A	L
A	G	A	P	E
T	A	P	I	R
A	L	E	R	T

Analock #5 — page 32

E	S	T	E	R
S	T	E	R	E
T	E	R	N	S
E	R	N	S	T
R	E	S	T	S

292

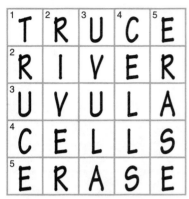

Analock #6   page 34

Analock #7   page 36

ALPHABETICS

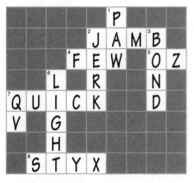

Alphabetic #1   page 46

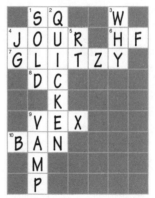

Alphabetic #2   page 48

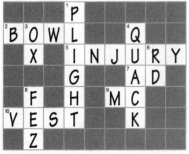

Alphabetic #3   page 50

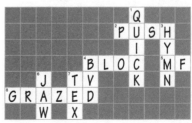

Alphabetic #4   page 52

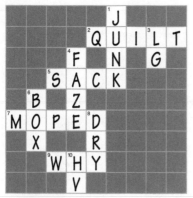

Alphabetic #5   page 54

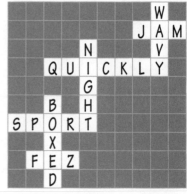

Alphabetic #6   page 56

NUMBER LOCKERS

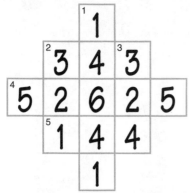

Number Locker #1   page 66

Number Locker #2   page 68

Number Locker #3   page 70

Number Locker #4   page 72

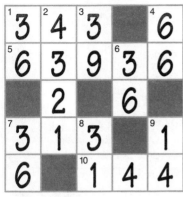

Number Locker #5   page 74

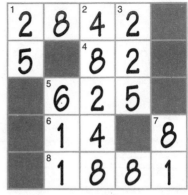

Number Locker #6   page 76

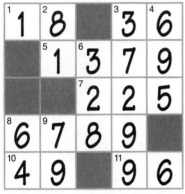

Number Locker #7   page 78

POSSIBLE PAIRS - *The "left brain" matches are all members of a single category or functionally related. The "right brain" matches are linked by a visual resemblance, metaphor, or pun.*

Left Brain Matches:
  mushroom — gravy boat
  angry man — Einstein
  hat — shoe
  tea kettle — tea cup
  light bulb — lamp
Right Brain Matches:
  mushroom — lamp
  angry man — tea kettle
  hat — tea cup
  shoe — gravy boat
  light bulb — Einstein

Possible Pair #1   page 86

Left Brain Matches:
  fat face — scared face
  VW — Cadillac
  stegosaurus — chicken
  "snail" pastry — pie
  beetle — snail

Right Brain Matches:
  fat face — pie
  VW — beetle
  "snail" pastry — snail
  scared face — chicken
  stegosaurus — Cadillac

Possible Pair #2   page 88

Left Brain Matches:
  ship — buoy
  crown — top hat
  baseball — boy
  camel — lion
  soap — bubbles
  chimney — smokestack
  cake — fork
Right Brain Matches:
  ship — camel
  crown — lion
  baseball — bubbles
  buoy — boy
  top hat — chimney
  fork — smokestack
  cake — (cake of) soap

Possible Pair #3   page 90

WORD WHEELS

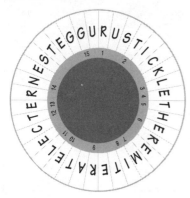

Word Wheel Intro   page 98

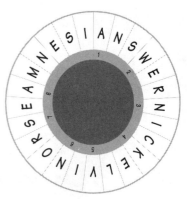

Word Wheel #1   page 102

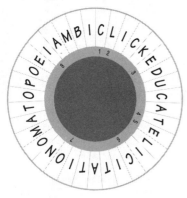

Word Wheel #2   page 104

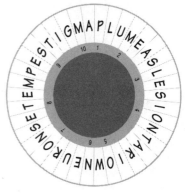

Word Wheel #3   page 106

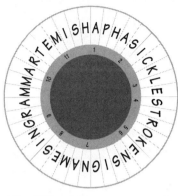

Word Wheel #4   page 108

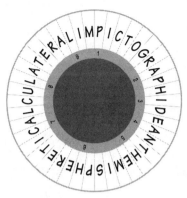

Word Wheel #5   page 110

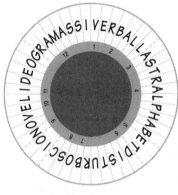

Word Wheel #6   page 112

Word Wheel #7   page 114

REAL-LIFE LOGIC

Betty had five suits and wore a different one each day of the workweek. The new shoes were worn every fourth day. Therefore, it was Monday of the fifth week (or the 21st day) before the combination came up again.

Logic #1   page 122

The five men brought in 75 fish. Harry caught 15 fish (half the 30 Jim caught), which was 20 percent of the total catch.

Logic #2   page 124

Adding $35 and $5 is purposeless. Dick has paid $45 for the two dinners, of which the cashier has $30, Dick has $10 returned to him, and the waiter has $5.

Logic #3   page 126

Able took an orange from the box labeled "Oranges and Grapefruit". Because *all* of the boxes were mislabeled, he knew that the box he drew from contained only oranges. He then relabeled the "Oranges and Grapefruit" box and switched the labels on the other two boxes.

Logic #4   page 128

Listing the first and second choices of each man, we have:

Tom: Able or Dismal
Dick: Better or Dismal
Harry: Better or
Jim: Better, Canny or Dismal

Tom made the right in selecting Able. Had one of the other three candidates been hired, he would have been the choice of more than one person.

Logic #5   page 130

ADDLOCKS

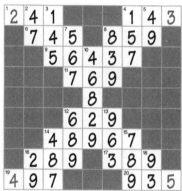

Addlock #1   page 142

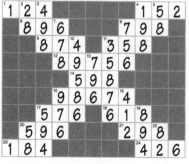

Addlock #2   page 144

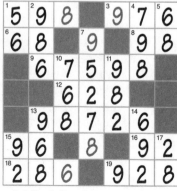

Addlock #3   page 146

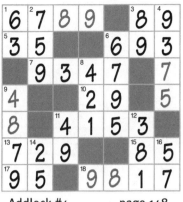

Addlock #4   page 148

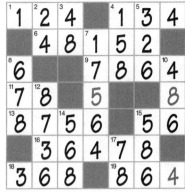

Addlock #5   page 150

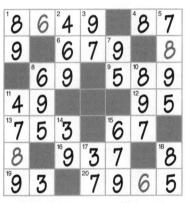

Addlock #6   page 152

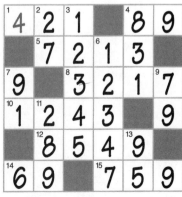

Addlock #7   page 154

Addlock #8   page 156

Addlock #9   page 158

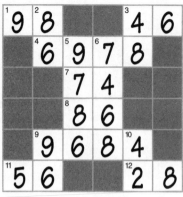

Addlock #10   page 160

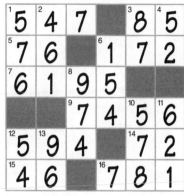

Addlock #11   page 162

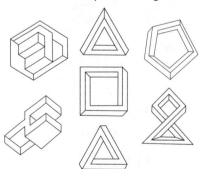

Addlock #12   page 164

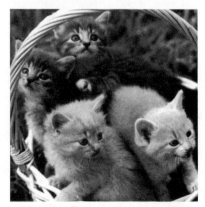

Addlock #13   page 166

LEFT-HEMI MEMORY

These are the "impossible" figures:

Memory #4   page 180

Memory #5   page 182

300

DIGI-CLUES

1	1	2	3
5	8	13	21
34	55	89	144

7	2	3	8	4
3	4	9	2	6
8	3	5	7	1
4	8	1	6	5
2	7	6	1	8

3	1	6	2	5
4	2	7	3	5
5	3	9	4	4
6	9	7	6	2
7	8	5	7	3

A	B	C
108	356	124
196	780	292
284	648	182

6	4	8	6	4
9	3	52	24	64
16	5	66	7	52

3	9	2	5	4
4	3	8	9	6
7	2	7	9	8
5	5	3	7	5
6	3	4	7	2

8	4	7
3	9	2
7	5	10
5	6	5

Digi-Clue #7   page 208

PROBLEMATICS

The chances are about even. Most people think that it's more likely to be a shop class, since shop classes generally have a majority of boys, and the class in question has a majority of boys. But note that 55% (the percentage of boys in this class) is halfway between 45% and 65% (the percentage of boys in home ec and shop classes in general), meaning, in effect, that the chances are about even of being one or the other.

Problematics #1   page 218

There will be about 72 families — the same number — with an order GBGGGG. You might think that the chances of having five girls and one boy would be less than those of having an even number of girls and boys, and you'd be right. But that's not the question. The question has to do with these particular sequences. Just as with lottery ticket numbers, any one sequence has the same chance of occurring as any other.

Problematics #2   page 220

The equal allocation — four to each family — is more likely than the seemingly more random allocation. To see how this must be so, imagine a similar situation involving just two families, and imagine a more extreme version of the slightly unequal distribution of 4-3-5-4-4. Imagine what would be in effect the logical extreme of an unequal distribution between two families, twenty yams given to one and none to the other, versus an equal allocation, ten and ten. Imagine further that the allocation-choosing procedure goes like this: randomly choose either one yam or none for one family, then one yam or none for the other, then go back to the first family and again choose one yam or none, then again with the second family, and so on until all the yams are exhausted. When the problem is presented this way, you can readily grasp that the chances of one family ending up with all the yams would be very small indeed compared to an even distribution.

Problematics #3   page 222

The reason why random-seeming number sequences are more frequently guessed is precisely because people expect a randomly-chosen number sequence to *appear* random. So the seemingly improved ability of listeners to guess some sequences relative to others says more about everyday human psychology than about parapsychological phenomena such as ESP.

Problematics #4   page 224

The mother chose, of course, to have her child born at the smaller hospital in Bandlapur. But she was wasting her time making the longer trip. The only reason the Bandlapur hospital had more days of the year on which at least 60% of births were boys was that it was smaller. With a smaller sample size, deviations from average are more likely.

Problematics #5   page 226

ANASEARCHES

ANASEARCH #1, page 234:
A. PAGES US, PEGASUS
B. SLICK PAST, SLAPSTICK
C. SPEND IT, STIPEND
D. REIN MARS, MARINERS
E. LAST TEE, SEATTLE
F. LENDS TREES, SLENDEREST
G. PRESETS, PESTERS
H. NEAR IT, RETAIN
I. BELT SUM, STUMBLE
J. VILE, EVIL
K. BANES, BEANS
L. LANES, LEANS
M. DAME, MEAD
N. SNIT, TINS
O. LASTED, SALTED
P. RESET, TERSE
Q. TIRE, RITE
R. REEL, LEER
S. NOTE, ETON

ANASEARCH #2, page 236:
A. BOAT AGES, SABOTAGE
B. TEEN'S CART, ENTR'ACTES
C. HAZY SCORER, CRAZY HORSE
D. CHARM, MARCH
E. ED VOTED, DEVOTED
F. RANTER, ERRANT
G. TO CUFF, CUT OFF
H. INN LAD, INLAND
I. MOON LAIR, MONORAIL
J. MONDE, DEMON
K. TALENT, LATENT
L. NAVE, VANE

ANASEARCH #3, page 238:
A. DANES, SNEAD
B. TONICS, TOCSIN
C. CANOE, OCEAN
D. STAR PROP, RAPPORTS
E. STIPEND, END PITS
F. MADDEN, DAMNED
G. REDRAW, REWARD
H. CALM, CLAM
I. GETAWAY, GATEWAY
J. MOST RUN, NOSTRUM
K. REPORTS, PORTERS
L. SWAGE, WAGES
M. SPURT IN, TURNIPS
N. REX MAINE, EXAMINER
O. NEWSTER, WESTERN
P. X-TREE, EXERT
Q. WE SING, SEWING
R. MAXI-O, AXIOM

ANASEARCH #4, page 240:
A. STORE UP, POSTURE
B. LINEN FROST, FRONTLINES
C. LEADER, REDEAL
D. STEAL, LEAST
E. LEAR, REAL
F. NUMBER, BEN RUM
G. TRAIL, TRIAL
H. LARK, KARL
I. TOWN HOUSE, SOUTH OWEN

M. SLOVEN, NOVELS
N. DAZE, ADZE
O. CLEAN, LANCE
P. REGAL, GLARE
Q. GOAT, TOGA

J. TRY PITCH, TRIPTYCH
K. END JASMINE, IN JAMES' DEN
L. ASTER, STARE
M. EGOS, GOES
N. MILES, LIMES
O. SECOND, ONE DSC
P. GEL SOT, LET'S GO
Q. MOON NOTE, MONOTONE
R. FACE, CAFE
S. STERN, NERTS

ANASEARCH #5, page 242:
A. TINGLES ON, SINGLETON
B. SPEAK YEAS, EASY PEAKS
C. STAND IT, DISTANT
D. FED IN BOUT, FINE DOUBT
E. AGREE, EAGER
F. SEE GRANT, ESTRANGE
G. I.E. RAP SAP, APPRAISE
H. REAL RUG, REGULAR
I. DARTS, STRAD
J. PRESTO, POSTER
K. COAL PIT, CAPITOL
L. DATE HOUR, AUTHORED
M. AUNT ST., TAUNTS
N. TRUST, STRUT
O. INFEST, FINEST
P. CANTS, SCANT
Q. SLIDE VASE, SEA DEVILS
R. READ, DEAR
S. OUGHTS, SOUGHT
T. ONE ST., STONE
U. A ROPE, OPERA

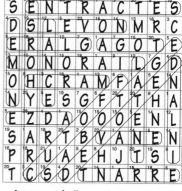

Anasearch #1   page 234

Anasearch #2   page 236

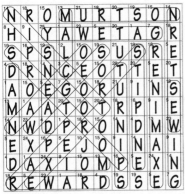

Anasearch #3   page 238

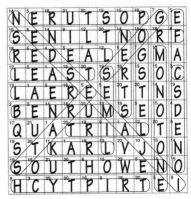

Anasearch #4   page 240

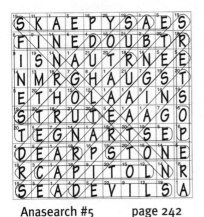

Anasearch #5   page 242

ALGEBRA GAMES

$$(11 \times 1) - 1 = 10$$
$$(2 \times 2 \times 2) + 2 = 10$$
$$(3 \times 3 \times 3 + 3) \div 3 = 10$$
$$(4 \times 4 + 4) \div \sqrt{4} = 10$$
$$5 + 5 = 10$$
$$[(6 + 6 \times 6) - (6 + 6)] \div 6 = 10$$
$$[(7 \times 7) + (7 + 7 + 7)] \div 7 = 10$$
$$[(8 \times 8) + (8 + 8)] \div 8 = 10$$
$$(9 \times 9 + 9) \div 9 = 10$$

Algebra Game #1   page 250

$$(7 + 7) \div (7 + 7) = 1$$
$$(7 \div 7) + (7 \div 7) = 2$$
$$7 + 7 + 7 \div 7 = 3$$
$$7 \times 7 - 7 \div 7 = 6$$
$$[(7 \times 7) + 7] \div 7 = 8$$
$$7 + 7 - (7 \div 7) = 13$$
$$(7 \div 7) + 7 + 7 = 15$$
$$(7 \times 7) - (7 \div 7) = 48$$
$$7 \times 7 + 7 - 7 = 49$$
$$[7 + (7 \div 7)] \times 7 = 56$$

Algebra Game #2   page 252

$$2 + 2 - 2 - 2 = 0$$
$$(2 \div 2) \times (2 \div 2) = 1$$
$$2 \div 2 + (2 \div 2) = 2$$
$$(2 + 2 + 2) \div 2 = 3$$
$$2 + 2 + 2 - 2 = 4$$
$$(2 \div 2) + 2 + 2 = 5$$
$$(2 \times 2 \times 2) - 2 = 6$$
$$[(2 \div .2) \div 2] + 2 = 7$$
$$(2 \times 2 \times 2) + 2 = 10$$
$$(2 + 2 + 2) \times 2 = 12$$

Algebra Game #3   page 254

$$(3+3+3) \div 3 = 3$$
$$[(3 \times 3)+3] \div 3 = 4$$
$$(3+3)-(3 \div 3) = 5$$
$$3+3+3-3 = 6$$
$$(3 \div 3)+3+3 = 7$$
$$(3 \times 3)-(3 \div 3) = 8$$
$$(3 \times 3)+3-3 = 9$$
$$(3 \times 3)+(3 \div 3) = 10$$

Algebra Game #4   page 256

$$(4+4) \div (4+4) = 1$$
$$(4 \times 4) \div (4+4) = 2$$
$$(4+4+4) \div 4 = 3$$
$$(4 \times 4) \div (\sqrt{4}+\sqrt{4}) = 4$$
$$[(4 \times 4)+4] \div 4 = 5$$
$$[(4 \times 4)-4] \div \sqrt{4} = 6$$
$$(4 \times \sqrt{4})-(4 \div 4) = 7$$
$$(4 \times 4)-(4+4) = 8$$
$$(4 \times \sqrt{4})+(4 \div 4) = 9$$
$$(4 \times \sqrt{4})+4-\sqrt{4} = 10$$

Algebra Game #5   page 258

MAGIC SQUARES

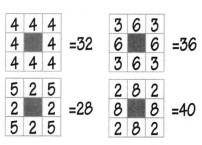

Magic Square #1   page 266

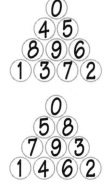

Magic Square #2   page 268

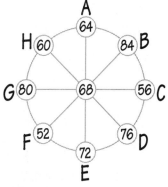

Magic Square #3   page 270

15	6	9	4
10	3	16	5
8	13	2	11
1	12	7	14

Magic Square #4   page 272

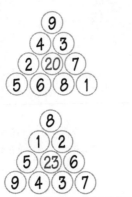

Magic Square #5   page 274

```
      2 + 0   = 2
      4 + 2   = 6
      6 + 4   = 1 0
  1 0 + 6   = 1 6
  1 6 + 1 0 = 2 6
  2 6 + 1 6 = 4 2
  4 2 + 2 6 = 6 8
  6 8 + 4 2 = 1 1 0
1 1 0 + 6 8 = 1 7 8
```

Codebreaker #1   page 282

```
      3 x 1 2 = 3 6
      9 x 4   = 3 6
  5 x 7 + 1 = 3 6
      1 8 x 2 = 3 6
      7 2 ÷ 2 = 3 6
      2 7 + 9 = 3 6
```

Codebreaker #2   page 284

```
      8 2 - 7 0 = 1 2
  1 2 + 6 - 3 = 1 5
      4 + 9 x 7 = 9 1
  9 x 8 - 1 5 = 5 7
  6 3 ÷ 7 + 8 = 1 7
      4 x 9 + 2 = 3 8
```

Codebreaker #3   page 286

```
  8 x 2 + 5 = 2 1
  4 x 5 x 6 = 1 2 0
  1 + 1 - 1 = 1
  1 + 1 x 8 = 1 6
  6 7 - 5 4 = 1 3
  3 x 6 + 7 = 2 5
```

Codebreaker #4   page 288

```
      8 + 9 = 1 7
  1 7 - 6 = 1 1
      6 x 5 = 3 0
      5 x 8 = 4 0
      3 x 7 = 2 1
      2 x 7 = 1 4
      9 x 5 = 4 5
```

Codebreaker #5   page 290

REFERENCES

Allen, L.S. and R.A. Gorski (1992). Sexual orientation and the size of the anterior commissure in the human brain. *Proceedings of the National Academy of Sciences USA* 89: 7199-7202.

Anaki, D., M. Faust, and S. Kravetz (1998). Cerebral hemispheric asymmetries in processing lexical metaphors. *Neuropsychologia* 36: 691-700.

Annett, M. and M.P. Alexander (1996). Atypical cerebral dominance: Predictions and tests of the right shift theory. *Neuropsychologia* 34: 1215-27.

Benbow, C.P. and D. Lubinski (1997). Psychological profile of the mathematically talented: Some sex differences and evidence supporting their biological basis. In M. Walsh (ed.), *Women, Men, and Gender*. New Haven: Yale University Press.

Bennett, E.L., M.R. Rosenzweig, M.C. Diamond, H. Morimoto, and M. Hebert (1974). Effects of successive environments on brain measures. *Physiology and Behavior* 12/4: 621-31.

Benton, A.L. (1980). The neuropsychology of facial recognition. *American Psychologist* 35: 176-86.

Bernstein, E.M. and F.W. Putnam (1986). Development, reliability, and validity of a dissociation scale. *The Journal of Nervous and Mental Disease* 174: 727-35.

Blum, D. (1997). *Sex on the Brain: The Biological Differences Between Men and Women*. New York: Penguin.

Bottini, G., et al. (1994). The role of the right hemisphere in the interpretation of figurative aspects of language: A positron emission tomography activation study. *Brain* 117: 1241-53.

Chiarello, C. (1988a). Lateralization of lexical processes in the normal brain: A review of visual half-field research. In H.A. Whitaker (ed.), *Contemporary Reviews in Neuropsychology*. New York: Springer.

Chiarello, C. (1988b). Semantic priming in the intact brain: Separate roles for the right and left hemispheres? In C. Chiarello (ed.), *Right Hemisphere Contributions to Lexical Semantics*. New York: Springer.

Coltheart, M., E. Hull, and D. Slater (1975). Sex differences in imagery and reading. *Nature* 253: 438-40.

Coren, S. (1995). Differences in divergent thinking as a function of handedness and sex. *American Journal of Psychology* 108/3: 311-25

Damasio, A. (1994). *Descartes' Error: Emotion, Reason, and the Human Brain*. New York: Avon.

Damasio, A. (1997). Towards a neuropathology of emotion and mood. *Nature* 386: 769-70.

Damasio, H., T. Grabowski, D. Tranel, R. Hichwa, and A. Damasio (1996). A neural basis for lexical retrieval. *Nature* 380: 499-505.

Dart, R.A. (1949). The predatory implement technique of Australopithecus. *American Journal of Physical Anthropology* 7: 1-38.

Davidson, R.J. and A.J. Tomarken (1989). Laterality and emotion: An electrophysiological approach. In F. Boller and J. Grafman (eds.), *Handbook of Neuropsychology*, volume 3. New York: Elsevier.

Dehaene, S. and L. Cohen (1997). Cerebral pathways for calculation: Double dissociations between Gerstmann's acalculia and subcortical acalculia. *Cortex* 33: 219-50.

Demb, J.B., et al. (1995). Semantic encoding and retrieval in the left inferior prefrontal cortex: A functional MRI study of task difficulty and process specificity. *Journal of Neuroscience* 15: 5870-78.

Démonet, J.-E., F. Chollet, S. Ramsay, D. Cardebat, J.-L. Nespoulous, R. Wise, A. Rascol, and R. Frackowiak (1992). The anatomy of phonological and semantic processing in normal subjects. *Brain* 115: 1753-68.

Diamond, M.C. (1988). *Enriching Heredity*. New York: Free Press.

Diamond, M.C. (1990). How the brain grows in response to experience. In R.E. Ornstein (ed.), *The Healing Brain: A Scientific Reader*. New York: Guilford.

Dimond, S.J., L. Farrington, and P. Johnson (1976). Differing emotional response from left and right hemispheres. *Nature* 261: 690-92.

Drake, R.A. and B.R. Bingham (1985). Induced lateral orientation and persuasibility. *Brain Cognition* 4: 156-64.

Edwards, B. (1989). *Drawing on the Right Side of the Brain*. Los Angeles: J.P. Tarcher.

Elias, L.J. and M.P. Bryden (in press). Footedness is a better predictor of language lateralization than handedness. *Laterality*.

Faust, M. and C. Chiarello (1998). Sentence context and lexical ambiguity resolution by the two hemispheres. *Neuropsychologia* 36: 827-35.

Gainotti, G. and C. Caltagirone (eds.) (1989). *Emotions and the dual brain*. Berlin/Heidelberg: Springer.

Gaulin, S.J.C. (1995). Does evolutionary theory predict sex differences in the brain? In M. Gazzaniga (ed.), *The Cognitive Neurosciences*. Cambridge, MA: MIT Press.

Gazzaniga, M.S. (1998). *The Mind's Past*. Berkeley: University of California Press.

Geschwind, N. and N. Galaburda (1987). *Cerebral Lateralization: Biological Mechanisms, Associations and Pathology*. Cambridge MA: MIT Press.

Goel, V., B. Bold, S. Kapur, and S. Houle (1998). Neuroanatomical correlates of human reasoning. *Journal of Cognitive Neuroscience* 10/3: 293-302.

Goldberg, E. (1990). Associative agnosias and the functions of the left hemisphere. *Journal of Clinical and Experimental Neuropsychology* 12: 467-84.

Goldberg, E. and L.D. Costa (1981). Hemispheric differences in the use and acquisition of descriptive systems. *Brain and Language* 14: 144-73.

Gur, R.C., R.E. Gur, W.D. Orbrist, J.P. Hungerbuhler, D. Younkin, A.D. Rosen, B.E. Skolnick, and M. Reivich (1982). Sex and handedness differences in cerebral blood flow during rest and cognitive activity. *Science* 217: 659-61.

Gur, R.E. and R.C. Gur (1990). Gender difference in regional cerebral blood flow. *Schizophrenia Bulletin* 16/2.

Gur, R.C., L.H. Mozley, P.D. Mozley, S.M. Resnick, J.S. Karp, A. Alavi, S.E. Arnold, and R.E. Gur (1995). Sex differences in regional cerebral glucose metabolism during a resting state. *Science* 267: 528-31.

Hampson, E. and D. Kimura (1988). Reciprocal effects of hormonal fluctuations on human motor and perceptual spatial skills. *Behavioural Neuroscience* 102/3: 456-9.

Hyde, J.S., E. Fennema, and S.J. Lamon (1990). Gender differences in mathematics performance: A meta-analysis. *Psychological Bulletin* 107: 139-55.

Hyman, I.E. and F.J. Billings (1998). Individual differences and the creation of false childhood memories. *Memory* 6/1: 1-20.

Inglis, J. and J.S. Lawson (1981). Sex differences in the effects of unilateral brain damage on intelligence. *Science* 212: 693-5.

Jaeger, J., A. Lockwood, D. Kemmerer, R. Van Valin, Jr., B.W. Murphy, and H, Khalak (1996). A positron emission tomographic study of regular and irregular verb morphology in English. *Language* 72/3: 451-97.

Jarvik, L.F. (1988). Aging of the brain: How can we prevent it? *The Gerontologist* 28: 739-47.

Kahneman, D. and A. Tversky (1972). Subjective probability: A judgment of representativeness. *Cognitive Psychology* 3: 430-54.

Kahneman, D. and C.A. Varey (1990). Propensities and counterfactuals: The loser that almost won. *Journal of Personality and Social Psychology* 59: 1101-1110.

Kapur, S., F.I.M. Craik, E. Tulving, A.A. Wilson, S. Houle, and G.M. Brown (1994). Neuroanatomical correlates of encoding in episodic memory: Levels of processing effect. *Proceedings of the National Academy of Science USA* 91: 2008-11.

Kimura, D. (1973). The asymmetry of the human brain. *Recent Progress in Perception*, March, 246-54.

Kimura, D. (1996). Sex, sexual orientation, and sex hormones influence human cognitive function. *Current Opinion in Neurobiology* 6: 259-63.

Kimura, D. and E. Hampson (1990). Neural and hormonal mechanisms mediating sex differences in cognition. *Research Bulletin* 689, Dept. of Psychology, University of Ontario, London, Canada.

Kinsbourne, M. (1983). Lateral input may shift activation balance in the integrated brain. *Psychologist* 38: 228-9.

Levick, S.E., T. Lorig, B.E. Wexler, R.E. Gur, R.C. Gur, and G.E. Schwartz (1993). Asymmetrical visual deprivation: A technique to differentially influence lateral hemispheric function. *Perceptual Motor Skills* 76: 1363-82.

Levy, J. (1990). The regulation and generation of perception in the asymmetric brain. In C. Trevarthen (ed.), *Brain Circuits and Functions of the Mind, Essays in Honor of Roger Sperry*. Cambridge: Cambridge University Press.

Levy, J. and M. Reid (1976). Variations in writing posture and cerebral organization. *Science* 194: 337.

Lezak, M.D. (1995). *Neuropsychological Assessment* (3rd edition). New York and Oxford: Oxford University Press.

Loftus, E.F. (1979). *Eyewitness Testimony*. Cambridge: Harvard University Press.

Loftus, E.F. and H.G. Hoffman (1989). Misinformation and memory: The creation of new memories. *The Journal of Experimental Psychology* 118/1: 100-4.

Loftus, E.F. and J.E. Pickrell (1995). The formation of false memories. *Psychiatric Annals* 25: 720-25.

McManus, I.C. and M.P. Bryden (1992). The genetics of handedness, cerebral dominance, and lateralization. In I. Rapin and S. Segalowitz (eds.), *Handbook of Neuropsychology*. New York: Elsevier.

Mikulincer, M., H. Babkoff, T. Caspy, and H. Sing (1989). The effects of 72 hours of sleep loss on psychological variables. *British Journal of Psychology* 80: 145-62.

Moffat, S.D. and E. Hampson (1996). A curvilinear relationship between testosterone and spatial cognition in humans: Possible influence of hand preference. *Psychoneuroendocrinology* 21: 323-37.

Nigro, G. and U. Neisser (1983). Point of view in personal memories. *Cognitive Psychology* 15: 467-82.

Oldfield, R.C. (1971). The assessment and analysis of handedness: The Edinburgh inventory. *Neuropsychologia* 9: 97-114.

Ornstein, R. (1997). *The Right Mind: Making Sense of the Hemispheres*. New York: Harcourt Brace and Company.

Pascual-Leone, A., M.D. Catalá, and A. Pascual-Leone Pascual (1996). Lateralized effect of rapid-rate transcranial magnetic stimulation of the prefrontal cortex on mood. *Neurology* 46/2: 499-502.

Petersen, S.E., P.T. Fox, A.Z. Snyder, and M.E. Raichle (1990). Activation of extrastriate and frontal cortical areas by visual words and word-like stimuli. *Science* 249: 1041-44.

Pettigrew, J.D. and S.M. Miller (1998). A "sticky" interhemispheric switch in bipolar disorder? Proceedings of the Royal Society of London Series B: *Biological Sciences* 265/1411: 2141-48.

Phelps, E.A. and M.S. Gazzaniga (1992). Hemispheric differences in mnemonic processing: The effects of left hemisphere interpretation. *Neuropsychologia* 30: 293-97.

Regard, M. and T. Landis (1988). Procedure vs. content learning: Effects of emotionality and repetition in a new clinical memory test. *Journal of Clinical and Experimental Neuropsychology* 10: 86.

Robertson, A.D. and J. Inglis (1977). Memory deficits after electroconvulsive therapy: Cerebral asymmetry and dual-encoding. *Neuropsychologia* 16: 179-87.

Robinson, J.A. and K.L. Swanson (1993). Field and observer modes of remembering. *Memory* 1: 169-84.

Rosenzweig, M.R., E.L. Bennett, and M.C. Diamond (1967). Effects of differential environments on brain anatomy and brain chemistry. *Proceedings of the Annual Meeting of the American Psychopathological Association* 56: 45-56.

Sackeim, H.A., M.S. Greenberg, A.L. Weiman, R.C. Gur, J.P. Hungerbuhler, and N. Geschwind (1982). Hemispheric asymmetry in the expression of positive and negative emotions: Neurological evidence. *Archives of Neurology* 39: 210-18.

Sagan, C. (1977). *The Dragons of Eden*. New York: Random House.

Sasanuma, M. and O. Fujimura (1971). Selective impairment of phonetic and non-phonetic transcription of words in Japanese aphasic patients: Kana vs. Kanji in visual recognition and writing. *Cortex* 7: 1-18.

Satz, P., D.L. Orsini, E. Saslow, and R. Henry (1985). The pathological left-handedness syndrome. *Brain and Cognition* 4: 27-46.

Schacter, D.L., E. Reiman, A. Uecker, M.R. Polster, L.S. Yun, and L.A. Cooper (1995). Brain regions associated with retrieval of structurally coherent visual information. *Nature* 376: 587-90.

Schacter, D.L. (1996). Searching for

Memory: *The Brain, the Mind, and the Past*. New York: BasicBooks.

Schiff, B. and M. Lamon (1994). Inducing emotion by unilateral contraction of hand muscles. *Cortex* 30: 247-54.

Schiffer, F. (1998). *Of Two Minds: The Revolutionary Science of Dual-Brain Psychology*. New York: The Free Press.

Shaywitz, B.A., S.E. Shaywitz, K.R. Pugh, R.T. Constable, P. Skudlarski, R.K. Fulbright, R.A. Bronen, J.M. Fletcher, D.P. Shakweiler, L. Katz, and J.C. Gore (1995). Sex differences in the functional organization of the brain for language. *Nature* 373: 607-8.

Smith, A. (1984). Early and long-term recovery from brain damage in children and adults: Evolution of concepts of localization, plasticity, and recovery. In C.E. Walker (ed.), *Handbook of clinical Psychology: Theory, Research, and Practice*. Homewood, IL: Dorsey Press.

Springer, S. and G. Deutsch (1998). *Left Brain, Right Brain: Perspectives from Cognitive Neuroscience*. New York: W.H. Freeman and Company.

Squire, L.R. (1992). Declarative and nondeclarative memory: Multiple brain systems supporting learning and memory. *Journal of Cognitive Neuroscience* 4: 232-43.

Stemmer, B. and F. Giroux (1994). Production and evaluation of requests by right hemisphere brain-damaged individuals. *Brain and Language* 47: 1-31.

Stromswold, K., D. Caplan, N. Alpert, and S. Rauch (1996). Localization of syntactic comprehension by Positron Emission Tomography. *Brain and Language* 52: 452-73.

Tulving, E. and D.M. Thomson (1973). Encoding specificity and retrieval processes in episodic memory. *Psychological Review* 80: 352-73.

Vargha-Khadem, F., E. Isaacs, and M. Mishkin (1994). Agnosia, alexia and a remarkable form of amnesia in an adolescent boy. *Brain* 117: 683-703.

Wilson, S.C. and T.X. Barber (1978). The Creative Imagination Scale as a measure of hypnotic responsiveness: Applications to experimental and clinical hypnosis. *American Journal of Clinical Hypnosis* 20: 235-49.

Winner, E. and H. Gardner (1977). The comprehension of metaphor in brain-damaged patients. *Brain* 100: 719-29.

Witelson, S. and D.L. Kigar (1992). Sylvian fissure morphology and asymmetry in men and women: Bilateral differences in relation to handedness in men. *Journal of Comparative Neurology* 323: 326-40.

Wittling, W. and M. Pflüger (1990). Neuroendocrine hemisphere asymmetries: Salivary cortisol secretion during lateralized viewing of emotion-related and neutral films. *Brain Cognition* 14: 243-65.

Wittling, W. and R. Roschmann (1993). Emotion-related hemisphere asymmetry: Subjective emotional responses to laterally presented films. *Cortex* 29: 431-48.

Zaidel, E. (1989). Language functions in the two hemispheres following complete cerebral commussurotomy and hemispherectomy. In F. Boller and J. Grafman (eds.), *Handbook of Neuropsychology*, volume 4. New York: Elsevier.

Zook, J.A. and J.H. Dwyer (1976). Cultural differences in hemisphericity: A critique. *Bulletin of the Los Angeles Neurological Societies* 41: 87-90.